I0702903

Thriving with Primary Biliary Cholangitis

A Healthy Diet Plan to Reduce Liver Workload, Support Bile Flow, and Manage PBC Symptoms| Includes Anti-Inflammatory Recipes and Liver Detox Tips

DR LANA BROWN, RN

Copyright Page

© 2024 by Dr. Lana Brown.

All rights reserved. No part of this cookbook may be reproduced, distributed, or transmitted in any form or by any means, including photocopying, recording, or other electronic or mechanical methods, without the prior written permission of the author, except in the case of brief quotations embodied in critical reviews and certain other noncommercial uses permitted by copyright law.

For permissions requests, write to the author at www.thelanabrown.com

Table of Contents

CHAPTER I

PRIMARY BILIARY CHOLANGITIS AND ITS IMPACT ON NUTRITION

Primary biliary cholangitis (PBC), formerly known as primary biliary cirrhosis, is an autoimmune disease in which the bile ducts are inflamed and slowly destroyed. These small channels carry the digestive fluid, or bile, from the liver to the small intestine. It previously was called primary biliary cirrhosis.

Bile is a fluid made in the liver. It helps with digestion and absorption of absorption of fat-soluble vitamins, such as A, D, E, and K.

It also helps the body absorb fats and get rid of cholesterol, toxins and worn-out red blood cells. Ongoing inflammation in the liver can lead to bile duct inflammation and damage known as cholangitis. At times, this can lead to permanent scarring of liver tissue, called cirrhosis. It also can eventually lead to liver failure.

Although it affects both sexes, primary biliary cholangitis mostly affects women. It's considered an autoimmune disease, which means your body's immune system is mistakenly attacking healthy cells and tissue. Researchers think a combination of genetic and environmental factors triggers the disease. It usually develops slowly.

"Cholangitis" means inflammation in your bile ducts. "Biliary" means of the bile ducts, and "primary" means original. This means that the disease itself is the original cause of inflammation in your bile ducts. There isn't some other condition causing inflammation, such as an infection or a blockage. Since the inflammation isn't responding to anything in particular, it doesn't know when to stop.

After their diagnosis, a person doesn't typically experience symptoms until 2 to 4.2 years later. However, some people may not have symptoms for over 17 years. And if a person has an earlier stage of PBC (stage 1 or 2), their life expectancy is average. However, everyone is different. Some people live longer than others with the disease. New treatments are improving the outlook for people with PBC.

At this time, there's no cure for primary biliary cholangitis, but medicines may slow liver damage, especially if treatment begins early.

What are the stages of primary biliary cholangitis?

PBC has four stages. They're based on how much damage has been done to the liver:

Stage 1: There's inflammation and damage to the walls of medium-sized bile ducts.

Stage 2: There's blockage of the small bile ducts.

Stage 3: This stage marks the beginning of scarring.

Stage 4: Cirrhosis has developed. This is permanent, severe scarring and damage to the liver.

Who does primary biliary cholangitis affect?

It primarily affects women and people assigned female at birth (AFAB), by a ratio of 10-to-1. In the U.S., it affects around 60 people AFAB per 100,000 and 15 people assigned male at birth (AMAB) per

100,000. Most are diagnosed after the age of 40. It's more common in Scotland, Scandinavia and Northeast England. It's also more common in people with a personal or family history of autoimmune disease, suggesting it might be a partly genetic disorder.

Symptoms

More than half of people with primary biliary cholangitis do not have any noticeable symptoms when diagnosed. The disease may be diagnosed when blood tests are done for other reasons, such as routine testing. Symptoms eventually develop over the next 5 to 20 years. Those who do have symptoms at diagnosis typically have poorer outcomes.

Common early symptoms include:

Fatigue.

Itchy skin.

Later signs and symptoms may include:

Yellowing of the skin and eyes, called jaundice.

Dry eyes and mouth.

Pain in the upper right abdomen.

Swelling of the spleen, called splenomegaly.

Bone, muscle or joint pain.

Swollen feet and ankles.

Buildup of fluid in the abdomen due to liver failure, called ascites.

Fatty deposits, called xanthomas, on the skin around the eyes, eyelids or in the creases of the palms, soles, elbows or knees.

Darkening of the skin that's not related to sun exposure, called hyperpigmentation.

Weak and brittle bones, called osteoporosis, which can lead to fractures.

High cholesterol.

Diarrhea that may include greasy stools, called steatorrhea.

Underactive thyroid, called hypothyroidism.

Weight loss.

Over time, your liver tissue can scar and harden. Other complications can start as the liver stops working because of scarring. This is called cirrhosis. Gallstones and bile duct stones can form, causing pain and infections.

These symptoms affect different people to different degrees. They can occur later or earlier in the course of your disease, and they can be mild to severe at any stage. How your symptoms present doesn't seem to be related to how advanced your disease is. However, some research has suggested that more severe symptoms earlier on may predict a faster progression overall.

Causes

It's not clear what causes primary biliary cholangitis. Many experts consider it an autoimmune disease in which the body turns against its own cells. Researchers believe this autoimmune response may be triggered by environmental and genetic factors.

The liver inflammation seen in primary biliary cholangitis starts when certain types of white blood cells called T cells, also known as T lymphocytes, start to collect in the liver. Usually, these immune cells detect and help defend against germs, such as bacteria and viruses. But in primary biliary cholangitis, they mistakenly destroy the healthy cells that line the small bile ducts in the liver.

Inflammation in the smallest ducts spreads and eventually damages other cells in the liver. As the cells die, they're replaced by scar tissue, also known as fibrosis, which can lead to cirrhosis. Cirrhosis is scarring of liver tissue that makes it difficult for your liver to work properly.

Risk factors

The following factors may increase your risk of primary biliary cholangitis:

Sex. Most people with primary biliary cholangitis are women.

Age. It's most likely to occur in people 30 to 60 years old.

Genetics. You're more likely to get the condition if you have a family member who has or had it.

Geography. It's most common in people of northern European descent, but primary biliary cholangitis can affect all ethnicities and races.

Researchers think that genetic factors combined with certain environmental factors trigger primary biliary cholangitis. These environmental factors may include:

Infections, such as a urinary tract infection.

Smoking cigarettes, especially over long periods of time.

Exposure to toxic chemicals, such as in certain work environments.

Complications

As liver damage worsens, primary biliary cholangitis can cause serious health problems, including:

Liver scarring, called cirrhosis. Cirrhosis makes it difficult for your liver to work and may lead to liver failure. It means the later stage of primary biliary cholangitis. People with primary biliary cholangitis and cirrhosis have a poor medical outlook. They also have a higher risk of other complications.

Jaundice. In jaundice, bile from the liver does not flow through the typical channels out of the liver and into the intestine. Instead, bile seeps into the bloodstream in higher than average amounts, causing a yellow hue in the eyes and skin.

Increased pressure in the portal vein, called portal hypertension. Blood from your intestine, spleen and pancreas enters your liver through a large blood vessel called the portal vein. When scar tissue from cirrhosis blocks normal blood flow through your liver, blood backs up. This causes increased pressure inside the vein. Also, because blood doesn't flow correctly through your liver, drugs and other toxins aren't filtered properly from your bloodstream.

Cholestasis. A major problem with PBC is cholestasis — when bile flow stops — within the liver, which causes the liver problems of PBC. However, cholestasis also leads to other problems when bile doesn't go to other parts of the body that need it to function properly, like the intestine and gallbladder.

Enlarged veins, called varices. When blood flow through the portal vein is slowed or blocked, blood may back up into other veins. It usually backs up into those in your stomach and esophagus. Increased pressure may cause delicate veins to break open and bleed. Bleeding in the upper stomach or esophagus is a life-threatening emergency. It requires immediate medical care.

Enlarged spleen, called splenomegaly. Your spleen may become swollen with white blood cells and platelets. This is because your body no longer filters toxins out of the bloodstream as it should.

Gallstones and bile duct stones. If bile cannot flow through the bile ducts, it may harden into stones in the ducts. These stones can cause pain and infection.

Liver cancer. Liver scarring increases your risk of liver cancer. If you have liver scarring, you'll need regular cancer screening.

Bone disease. About 30% of people with PBC experience mild changes in bone density known as osteopenia. Another 10% experience significant bone density losses enough to cause osteoporosis. It's likely that people with PBC experience bone changes because cholestasis associated with PBC means there's less bile in the intestines. This lack of bile in the intestines contributes to vitamin deficiency (A, D, E, K) in your body, since bile helps your body absorb these vitamins. One consequence is reduced bone health because vitamin D deficiency is related to low bone density.

Vitamin deficiencies. Not having enough bile affects your digestive system's ability to absorb fats and the fat-soluble vitamins, A, D, E and K. Because of this, some people with advanced primary biliary cholangitis may have low levels of these vitamins. Low levels can result in a variety of health problems, including night blindness and bleeding disorders.

High cholesterol. Up to 80% of people with primary biliary cholangitis have high cholesterol.

Decreased mental function, called hepatic encephalopathy. Some people with advanced primary biliary cholangitis and cirrhosis have personality changes. They also may have problems with memory and concentration.

Increased risk of other disease. Primary biliary cholangitis is associated with other disorders, including those that affect the thyroid, skin and joints. It also can be associated with dry eyes and mouth, a disorder called Sjogren's syndrome.

Diagnosis

Your healthcare professional will ask you about your health history and your family's health history, and perform a physical exam. The following tests and procedures may be used to diagnose primary biliary cholangitis.

Blood tests:

• **Liver tests**. These blood tests check the levels of certain proteins that may signal liver disease and bile duct injury.

• **Antibody tests for signs of autoimmune disease**. Blood tests may be done to check for anti-mitochondrial antibodies, also known as AMAs. These substances almost never occur in people without the disease, even if they have other liver disorders. Therefore, a positive AMA test is considered a very reliable sign of the disease.

However, a small number of people with primary biliary cirrhosis don't have AMAs.

• **Cholesterol test**. More than half the people with primary biliary cholangitis have extreme increases in blood fats, including total cholesterol level.

Imaging tests may help your healthcare team confirm a diagnosis or rule out other conditions with similar signs and symptoms. Imaging tests looking at the liver and bile ducts may include:

• **Ultrasound.** Ultrasound uses high-frequency sound waves to produce images of structures inside your body.

• **FibroScan.** Using an ultrasound-like probe, this test can detect scarring of the liver.

•**Magnetic   resonance cholangiopancreatography**, also known as

MRCP. This special MRI creates detailed images of your organs and bile ducts.

• **Magnetic resonance elastography**, also known as MRE. MRI is combined with sound waves to create a visual map of internal organs, called an elastogram. The test is used to detect hardening of your liver that might be a sign of cirrhosis.

If the diagnosis is still uncertain, your healthcare professional may perform a liver biopsy. A small sample of liver tissue is removed through an incision using a thin needle. It's then tested in a lab, either to confirm the diagnosis or to determine the extent of the disease.

Treatment

Treating the disease

There's no cure for primary biliary cholangitis, but medicines are available to help slow the progression of the disease and prevent complications. Options include:

• **Ursodeoxycholic acid**. This medicine, also known as UDCA or ursodiol (Actigall, Urso), is commonly used first. It helps move bile through your liver. UDCA doesn't cure primary biliary cholangitis, but it seems to improve liver function and reduce liver scarring. It's less likely to help with itching and fatigue. Side effects may include weight gain, hair loss and diarrhea.

• **Obeticholic acid (Ocaliva)**. Studies show that when obeticholic acid is given alone or combined with ursodiol for 12 months, it can help improve liver function and slow liver fibrosis. However, its use is often limited because it can cause increased itching.

• **Fibrates (Tricor)**. Researchers aren't exactly sure how this medicine works to help ease primary biliary cholangitis symptoms. But, when taken with UDCA, it has reduced liver inflammation and itching in some people. More studies are needed to determine long-term benefits.

• **Budesonide.** When combined with UDCA, the corticosteroid budesonide may be of potential benefit for primary biliary cholangitis. However, this medicine is associated with steroid-related side effects for people with more advanced disease. More long-term trials are necessary before budesonide can be recommended for treating this condition.

• **Liver transplant**. When medicines no longer control primary biliary cholangitis and the liver begins to fail, a liver transplant may help prolong life. A liver transplant replaces your diseased liver with a healthy one from a donor. Liver transplantation is associated with very good long-term outcomes for people with primary biliary cholangitis. However, sometimes the disease comes back several years later in the transplanted liver.

Treating the symptoms

Your healthcare team may recommend treatments to control the signs and symptoms of primary biliary cholangitis and make you more comfortable.

Treatment for fatigue

Primary biliary cholangitis causes fatigue. But your daily habits, proper diet and exercise, and other health conditions can affect how tired you feel. It is important to also be tested to exclude thyroid disease since it is more common in people with primary biliary cholangitis.

Treatment for itching

• **Antihistamines** are commonly used to reduce itching. They may help with sleep if itching keeps you awake. Antihistamines may include diphenhydramine, hydroxyzine hydrochloride and loratadine.

• **Cholestyramine** is a powder that may stop itching. It must be mixed with food or liquids.

• **Rifampin** is an antibiotic that may stop itching. Exactly how it does this is unknown. Researchers think it may block the brain's response to itch-inducing chemicals in the blood.

• **Opioid antagonists** such as those containing naloxone and naltrexone may help itching related to liver disease. Like rifampin, these medicines seem to reduce the itching sensation by acting on your brain.

• **Sertraline** is a medicine that increases serotonin in the brain, called a selective serotonin reuptake inhibitor, or SSRI. It can help reduce itching.

Treatment for dry eyes and mouth

Artificial tears and saliva substitutes can help ease dry eyes and mouth. They may be available with or without a prescription. Chewing gum or sucking on hard candy also can help you make more saliva and relieve dry mouth.

Treating the complications

Certain complications are commonly associated with primary biliary cholangitis. Your healthcare team may recommend:

• **Vitamin and mineral supplements**. If your body isn't absorbing vitamins or other nutrients, you may need to take vitamins A, D, E and K. You also may need calcium, folic acid or iron supplements.

• **Medicine to lower cholesterol**. If you have high cholesterol levels in your blood, your healthcare team may recommend taking a medicine known as a statin to help lower your levels.

• **Medicines to treat bone loss.** If you have weak or thinning bones, called osteoporosis, you may be prescribed medicines or supplements, such as calcium and vitamin D, to reduce bone loss and improve bone density. Exercise such as walking and using light weights most days of the week can help increase your bone density.

• **Treatment for increased pressure in the portal vein, called portal hypertension**. Your healthcare team is likely to screen and monitor you for portal hypertension and enlarged veins if you have more advanced scarring from liver disease. Fluid in your abdomen is a common side effect of portal hypertension. For mild fluid in the abdomen, your healthcare team may only recommend limiting salt in your diet. More-severe cases may require medicines known as diuretics or a procedure to drain the fluid called paracentesis.

The Liver's Role in Digestion and Metabolism

The liver is a large, wedge-shaped organ located in the upper right quadrant of the abdomen. It consists of two main lobes, divided into smaller lobes called lobules. The liver receives dual blood supply from the hepatic artery and the portal vein. The hepatic artery supplies oxygenated blood, while the portal vein delivers nutrient-rich blood from the gastrointestinal tract.

Metabolic Functions of the Liver:

The liver plays a central role in metabolism, contributing to various processes that are crucial for maintaining homeostasis in the body. Here are key metabolic functions of the liver:

• **Carbohydrate Metabolism**: The liver is involved in glycogen synthesis and storage, as well as glycogenolysis, the breakdown of glycogen into glucose. It also participates in gluconeogenesis, the synthesis of glucose from non-carbohydrate sources, ensuring a steady supply of glucose for energy production.

• **Lipid Metabolism**: The liver is responsible for the synthesis of cholesterol, bile acids, and phospholipids. It also plays a vital role in lipid metabolism by converting excess dietary carbohydrates into triglycerides for storage or transport in the bloodstream.

• **Protein Metabolism:** The liver is involved in protein synthesis and degradation. It synthesizes important plasma proteins, such as albumin, clotting factors, and complement proteins. It also plays a role in the urea cycle, which eliminates toxic ammonia produced during protein metabolism.

• **Drug Metabolism**: The liver metabolizes drugs and toxins, transforming them into more water-soluble compounds for excretion. This detoxification process involves enzymatic reactions mediated by liver enzymes, such as the cytochrome P450 system.

Digestive Function of the Liver:

• **Producing important substances**. Your liver continually produces bile. This is a chemical that helps turn fats into energy that your body uses. Bile is necessary for the digestive process. Your liver also creates albumin. This is a blood protein that helps carry hormones, drugs, and fatty acids throughout your body. Your liver also creates most of the substances that help your blood clot after injury.

Importance of Nutrition in Managing PBC

Nutrition is really important when it comes to managing Primary Biliary Cholangitis (PBC), a chronic liver disease caused by the immune system attacking the bile ducts. Here's why prioritizing an healthy diet matters so much:

1. Supporting Your Liver: A balanced diet helps keep your liver as healthy as possible. Since PBC affects the bile ducts inside your liver, eating right can help manage symptoms and slow down the disease.

2. Getting Essential Nutrients: PBC can mess with how your body absorbs vitamins like A, D, E, and K. Eating a balanced diet ensures you're getting enough of these nutrients, either from food or supplements.

3. Boosting Energy Levels: Fatigue is a big issue for people with PBC. Eating well gives you the energy you need to fight fatigue and stay active.

4. Maintaining a Healthy Weight: PBC can make your weight go up and down. Eating a balanced diet helps you keep a healthy weight, which is important for your liver and overall health.

5. Reducing Inflammation: Some foods can make liver inflammation worse. A good diet can help calm inflammation and ease symptoms.

6. Supporting Your Medications: The meds you take for PBC might work better if you're eating right. Your diet can affect how well your meds work, so it's important to follow a good eating plan.

7. Managing Symptoms: Eating the right foods can help with symptoms like fluid retention or digestive issues that come with PBC.

8. Overall Well-Being: Good nutrition supports your immune system and keeps you healthier overall, which is super important when you're dealing with a chronic condition like PBC.

CHAPTER II

DIETARY GUIDELINES FOR MANAGING PBC

General Diet Principles for PBC Patients

Although there is no single diet for PBC, there are still many dietary recommendations for individuals with PBC.

Modified Mediterranean Diet

Because PBC is an inflammatory condition, an anti-inflammatory diet, such as the Mediterranean diet, is recommended. This should be modified to meet individual needs.

The Mediterranean diet is essentially a healthy, well-balanced diet that emphasizes whole plant-based foods and healthy fats. It is a diet rich in fruits and vegetables (at least servings), as well as unsaturated fats, lean meats, whole grains, and complex carbohydrates. Proper nutrition throughout all stages of PBC helps the liver to function at its best.

Mixed Recommendations on Coffee

A registered dietitian working at a transplant center in Chicago advises individuals with PBC to drink coffee without sugar or cream if they can tolerate it due to evidence supporting coffee's ability to reduce the risk of liver cancer. In contrast, PBCers Organization recommends the avoidance or limited consumption of caffeine.

Foods to Avoid or Reduce

Several sources agree that people with PBC should do the following:

Avoid foods high in sugar, (sugar-sweetened beverages, high-fructose corn syrup, sodas, and fruit drinks) because consumption of sugary foods that are absorbed by the liver may lead to fatty liver disease.

Avoid foods high in saturated fats, such as dairy products, beef and pork with visible fat, and processed meats, and consume a low-fat diet because individuals with PBC have trouble absorbing fats due to decreased bile availability, potentially leading to diarrhea and weight loss; however, it is important to eat healthy fats as a part of a balanced diet and not eliminate fats completely.

Reduce sodium intake, and cook with salt-free seasoning blends.

Completely avoid or limit consumption of alcohol, (particularly in individuals with PBC-related cirrhosis).

Avoid foods that may increase the risk of foodborne illness, including raw or undercooked meat, fish, shellfish, and unpasteurized milk products, as individuals with PBC are more susceptible to developing severe bacterial or viral infections from these foods.

Dietary Fat Modification

Patients with PBC who have insufficient bile acids in the small intestine as evidenced by increased fat excretion in the stool (steatorrhea) due to fat malabsorption can make dietary modifications that may reduce these manifestations. It is recommended to substitute dietary medium-chain triglycerides, such as coconut oil and dairy, for long-chain triglycerides, such as nuts, avocados, and meat, and reduce total fat intake.

Eating Smaller Meals

Eating smaller meals more frequently throughout the day (around 4 to small meals per day) can help the liver process food and toxins more efficiently and easily.

Low-Sodium Diet

Individuals in the advanced stages of PBC with ascites, peripheral edema, or other signs and symptoms of fluid overload may require a low-sodium diet to avoid further fluid retention.

Diets for Gaining Weight

Individuals with advanced liver disease may also experience significant weight loss due to nausea and poor appetite. Candidates for liver transplantation may need to gain weight to optimize surgical outcomes.

Protein-energy malnourishment is often observed in individuals with end-stage liver disease before they undergo liver transplantation. Pretransplant loss of skeletal lean muscle mass (sarcopenia) can be significantly detrimental to post-transplant outcomes.

Micronutrient Considerations (Vitamins and Minerals)

Individuals with PBC are at risk for fat-soluble vitamin deficiency and may not be able to meet these nutritional needs from dietary sources alone. Testing and consultation with a care team is essential before initiating supplementation;

however, physicians and dieticians can help prepare a plan including supplementation with fat-soluble vitamins A, D, E, or K if deficiencies are present. Dietary supplements are not regulated by the US Food and Drug Administration (FDA), so it is important to follow doctor recommendations as to the quantity and type of supplements to ensure adequate supplementation.

According to the National Institute of Diabetes and Digestive and Kidney Diseases (NIDDK), if individuals with PBC are at risk of developing osteoporosis, physicians may recommend eating foods high in calcium and vitamin D or take these dietary supplements to prevent osteoporosis.

Fluid Intake Recommendations

When managing primary biliary cholangitis (PBC), a chronic liver condition, it's essential to focus on staying well-hydrated to support liver function. Here are some practical tips:

1. Stay Hydrated: Make sure you drink enough fluids throughout the day to keep yourself hydrated. Water is the best choice for this.

2. Choose Water: Aim to drink water regularly. It helps maintain hydration levels and supports overall health.

3. Limit Sugary Drinks and Alcohol: It's best to cut down on sugary beverages and avoid alcohol, as both can strain the liver.

4. Moderate Caffeine: Enjoy coffee or tea in moderation. Small amounts of caffeine can be okay, but excessive intake should be avoided.

6. Watch Sodium Intake: If you're prone to fluid retention, keep an eye on your sodium intake. It can help manage any swelling.

7. Personalized Advice: Since PBC affects everyone differently, it's important to get personalized advice from your healthcare provider or a liver specialist. They can tailor recommendations to your specific needs and health status.

Chapter 3: Foods and Substances to Avoid

Impact of Alcohol on Liver Health

Alcohol can really affect your liver health, mainly through something called alcoholic liver disease (ALD). Your liver's job is to process alcohol, and if you drink a lot over time, it can lead to serious problems:

1. Fatty Liver: This happens first when fat builds up in your liver cells. It can get better if you stop drinking early on.

2. Alcoholic Hepatitis: This is when your liver gets inflamed from too much alcohol. It can range from feeling uncomfortable to being really sick, with symptoms like yellow skin (jaundice), fever, and belly pain. It needs medical attention because it can be life-threatening.

3. Cirrhosis: This is the worst stage of ALD, where your liver gets scarred permanently. It messes up how your liver works and can lead to liver failure. You might get a big belly from fluid buildup (ascites), feel confused (hepatic encephalopathy), and have more infections or bleeding problems.

4. Liver Cancer: Drinking a lot over time also raises your chance of getting liver cancer, especially if you already have cirrhosis.

How alcohol affects your liver depends on how much you drink and for how long. Things like your genes and overall health also matter.

To keep your liver safe:

- **Moderate Drinking:** Stick to no more than one drink a day for women or two for men.

- **Avoid Bingeing:** Drinking a lot in a short time is really hard on your liver.

- **Get Checked**: If you drink a lot or think you might have liver issues, see your doctor regularly.

Potential Harmful Food Additives and Medications

When dealing with primary biliary cholangitis (PBC), a chronic liver condition, it's important to be mindful of certain food additives and medications that could potentially harm your liver. Here are some things to watch out for:

Harmful Food Additives:

1. **Artificial Sweeteners**: Some studies suggest artificial sweeteners like those in diet sodas might not be great for liver health.

2. **Trans Fats:** These are found in a lot of processed foods and can contribute to liver problems.

3. **High Fructose Corn Syrup:** It's in many sugary drinks and processed foods and can also cause liver issues.

4. **Food Dyes and Preservatives**: Some of these additives have been linked to liver damage in some people.

Medications to Be Cautious About:

1. **Certain Antibiotics:** Some antibiotics can affect the liver, so it's important to use them carefully if you have PBC.

2. Non-Steroidal Anti-Inflammatory Drugs (NSAIDs): Pain relievers like ibuprofen and naproxen can be tough on your liver, so use them only when necessary.

3. Statins: These are used to lower cholesterol but can sometimes affect liver enzymes. Your doctor may monitor you closely if you're on statins.

4. Immunosuppressants: If you're taking these for another condition, they might need adjustments because they can also impact your liver.

When dealing with primary biliary cholangitis (PBC), a chronic liver condition, it's important to be mindful of certain food additives and medications that could potentially harm your liver. Here are some things to watch out for:

Harmful Food Additives:

1. **Artificial Sweeteners**: Some studies suggest artificial sweeteners like those in diet sodas might not be great for liver health.

2. **Trans Fats:** These are found in a lot of processed foods and can contribute to liver problems.

3. **High Fructose Corn Syrup:** It's in many sugary drinks and processed foods and can also cause liver issues.

4. **Food Dyes and Preservatives**: Some of these additives have been linked to liver damage in some people.

Medications to Be Cautious About:

1. **Certain Antibiotics**: Some antibiotics can affect the liver, so it's important to use them carefully if you have PBC.

2. Non-Steroidal Anti-Inflammatory Drugs (NSAIDs): Pain relievers like ibuprofen and naproxen can be tough on your liver, so use them only when necessary.

3. Statins: These are used to lower cholesterol but can sometimes affect liver enzymes. Your doctor may monitor you closely if you're on statins.

4. Immunosuppressants: If you're taking these for another condition, they might need adjustments because they can also impact your liver.

High-Cholesterol and Effect on Liver Function

You've probably heard that eating too much cholesterol is bad for your heart. But it may be even worse for your liver.

Cholesterol from food mostly ends up in the liver. If you are getting too much, this can increase your risk for fatty liver disease. High cholesterol also can turn fatty liver disease (steatosis) into a more serious and sometimes fatal condition known as nonalcoholic steatohepatitis (NASH).

 When fatty liver disease turns into NASH, it can lead to other liver problems including:

Liver inflammation

Scarring (cirrhosis)

Liver failure

Liver cancer

Changes in lipids including cholesterol also may play a role in other chronic liver diseases, including:

Alcoholic liver disease

Hepatitis C

Hepatitis B

Cholestatic liver disease

Cirrhosis

Managing Cholesterol to Protect Your Liver

If you have high cholesterol and concerns about your liver, there's a lot you can do to reduce your risks and protect your liver. These steps include:

- Getting regular aerobic exercise

- Eating less saturated or trans fat
- Eating more fiber
- Eating fewer carbohydrates
- Maintaining a healthy weight

Studies have shown that a Mediterranean diet is good for your liver. A Mediterranean diet includes lower amounts of red meat and dairy and is rich in:

Vegetables

Fruits

Whole grains

Beans

Nuts and seeds

Olive oil

If you have liver disease and diet and exercise aren't enough to lower your cholesterol, your doctor may suggest you take a cholesterol-lowering medicine. Doctors most often prescribe statins for this.

If you have high cholesterol and think your liver may be at risk, talk to your doctor about steps you can take to lower your risks.

Other Substances to Limit or Avoid

Avoid saturated fats like cream and butter and cut back or eliminate beef and pork with visible fat, sausages, bacon and deli meats. Always remember: fats are part of a balanced diet and should not be avoided completely. It's true that people with PBC often have problems absorbing fats and fat-soluble vitamins because they have less bile. The undigested fats can cause diarrhea, weight loss and other complications. As a result, sometimes PBC patients think they should drastically reduce all fats. That's a mistake. The key is to eat healthy fats.

Stay away from foods high in sugar, especially sugar-sweetened beverages such as sodas, fruit drinks, and high fructose corn syrup. Here's why: when the liver is forced to absorb too much sugar, it leads to fatty deposits that can eventually build up and result in fatty liver disease (newly renamed to steatotic liver disease). On the other hand, don't refrain from the naturally occurring sugar in fruits, which are great for people with PBC.

Reduce sodium. If you have edema or ascites, cutting back on sodium is extremely important. But even if you don't have those symptoms, you should get your sodium intake under control. Start by avoiding the salt shaker at the dinner table. Cook with seasonings that do not contain any sodium such as salt-free blends (e.g, Mrs. Dash). I don't want to suggest a specific amount of sodium, as diets will vary and there are variations in low- and moderate-sodium diets.

CHAPTER IV

NOURISHING BREAKFAST RECIPES FOR PBC

Delicious Vegetable Omelets

Ingredients

• ½ cup no-salt-added diced tomatoes with basil, garlic, and oregano, well drained

• ½ cup cucumber, chopped and seeded

• ½ cup chopped yellow summer squash

• ½ ripe avocado, pitted, peeled, and chopped

• 2 eggs

• 1 cup refrigerated or frozen egg product, thawed

• 2 tablespoons water

• 1 teaspoon dried basil, crushed

• ¼ teaspoon salt

• ¼ teaspoon ground black pepper

• Nonstick cooking spray

• ¼ cup shredded reduced-fat Monterey Jack cheese with jalapeño chile peppers

• 1 Snipped fresh chives

Directions

1. For filling, in a medium bowl stir together tomatoes, cucumber, squash and avocado. Set aside. In a medium bowl whisk together eggs, egg product, water, basil, salt and pepper.

2. For each omelet, coat an 8-inch nonstick skillet generously with cooking spray. Heat skillet over medium heat. Add a generous 1/3 cup of the egg mixture to hot skillet.

3. Immediately begin stirring eggs gently but continuously with a wooden spatula until mixture resembles cooked egg pieces surrounded by liquid egg. Stop stirring. Cook for 30 to 60 seconds more or until egg is set but shiny.

4. Spoon 1/2 cup of the filling over one side of omelet. Carefully fold omelet over the filling. Very carefully remove omelet from skillet. Repeat to make 4 omelets total, using paper towels to wipe skillet clean and spraying with cooking spray between omelets. Sprinkle 1 tablespoon of cheese over each omelet. If desired, garnish with chives.

Tomato-&-Avocado Cheese Sandwich

Ingredients

• 2 slices whole-wheat bread

• ¼ avocado, mashed

• 3 slices tomato

• ¼ cup grated Parmesan cheese

• 1 cup mixed salad greens or baby spinach

• 2 teaspoons balsamic vinegar

• 1 medium ripe pear

Directions

1. Lay bread on work surface. Spread avocado on one slice. Top with tomatoes and sprinkle with cheese. Toast both pieces of bread in a toaster oven

until the plain piece is toasted and the cheese is starting to melt on the topped piece, 4 to 6 minutes.

2. Remove the toast from the toaster oven with a spatula, and mound greens (or spinach) on top of the cheese side. Drizzle with vinegar and top with the remaining toast. Cut in half if desired and serve with pear.

Spinach & Egg Scramble with Raspberries

Ingredients

• 1 teaspoon canola oil

• 1 ½ cups baby spinach (1 1/2 ounces)

• 2 large eggs, lightly beaten

• Pinch of kosher salt

- Pinch of ground pepper

- 1 slice whole-grain bread, toasted

- ½ cup fresh raspberries

Directions

1. Heat oil in a small nonstick skillet over medium-high heat. Add spinach and cook until wilted, stirring often, 1 to 2 minutes. Transfer the spinach to a plate. Wipe the pan clean, place over medium heat and add eggs. Cook, stirring once or twice to ensure even cooking, until just set, 1 to 2 minutes. Stir in the spinach, salt and pepper. Serve the scramble with toast and raspberries.

Fig & Ricotta Overnight Oats

Ingredients

- ½ cup old-fashioned rolled oats

- ½ cup water

- Pinch of salt

- 2 tablespoons part-skim ricotta cheese

- 2 tablespoons chopped dried figs

- 1 tablespoon toasted sliced almonds

- 2 teaspoons honey

Directions

1. Combine oats, water and salt in a jar or bowl and stir. Cover and refrigerate overnight.

2. In the morning, heat the oats, if desired, or eat cold. Top with ricotta, figs, almonds and honey.

Blueberry-Banana Overnight Oats

Ingredients

- ½ cup unsweetened coconut milk beverage

- ½ cup old-fashioned oats

- ½ tablespoon chia seeds (Optional)

- ½ banana, mashed

- 1 teaspoon maple syrup

- Pinch of salt

- ½ cup fresh blueberries

- 1 tablespoon unsweetened flaked coconut (Optional)

Directions

1. Combine coconut milk, oats, chia seeds (if using), banana, maple syrup and salt in a pint-sized jar and stir. Top with blueberries and coconut, if desired. Cover and refrigerate overnight.

Easy Loaded Baked Omelet Muffins

Ingredients

• 3 slices bacon, chopped

• 2 cups finely chopped broccoli

• 4 scallions, sliced

• 8 large eggs

• 1 cup shredded Cheddar cheese

• ½ cup low-fat milk

• ½ teaspoon salt

• ½ teaspoon ground pepper

Directions

1. Preheat oven to 325 degrees F. Coat a 12-cup muffin tin with cooking spray.

2. Cook bacon in a large skillet over medium heat until crisp, 4 to 5 minutes. Remove with a slotted spoon to a paper towel-lined plate, leaving the bacon fat in the pan. Add broccoli and scallions and cook, stirring, until soft, about 5 minutes. Remove from heat and let cool for 5 minutes.

3. Meanwhile, whisk eggs, cheese, milk, salt and pepper in a large bowl. Stir in the bacon and broccoli mixture. Divide the egg mixture among the prepared muffin cups.

4. Bake until firm to the touch, 25 to 30 minutes. Let stand for 5 minutes before removing from the muffin tin.

Tasty Fig & Ricotta Toast

Ingredients

• 1 slice crusty whole-grain bread (1/2-inch thick)

• ¼ cup part-skim ricotta cheese

• 1 fresh fig or 2 dried, sliced

• 1 teaspoon sliced almonds, toasted

• 1 teaspoon honey

• Pinch of flaky sea salt, such as Maldon

Directions

1. Toast bread. Top with ricotta cheese, figs and almonds. Drizzle with honey and sprinkle with sea salt.

Goat Cheese, Blackberry and Almond Topped Toast

Ingredients

- ½ ounce goat cheese (chèvre)

- 1 slice 100% whole wheat bread, lightly toasted

- 2 tablespoons blackberries

- 1 tablespoon sliced almonds

- 1 teaspoon honey

Directions

1. Spread goat cheese on toast. Top with blackberries and almonds. Drizzle with honey.

Baked Banana-Nut Oatmeal Cups

Ingredients

• 3 cups rolled oats

• 1 ½ cups low-fat milk

• 2 ripe bananas, mashed (about 3/4 cup)

• ⅓ cup packed brown sugar

• 2 large eggs, lightly beaten

• 1 teaspoon baking powder

• 1 teaspoon ground cinnamon

• 1 teaspoon vanilla extract

• ½ teaspoon salt

• ½ cup toasted chopped pecans

Directions

1. Preheat oven to 375°F. Coat a muffin tin with cooking spray.

2. Combine oats, milk, bananas, brown sugar, eggs, baking powder, cinnamon, vanilla and salt in a large bowl. Fold in pecans. Divide the mixture among the muffin cups (about 1/3 cup each). Bake until a toothpick inserted in the center comes out clean, about 25 minutes. Cool in the pan for 10 minutes, then turn out onto a wire rack. Serve warm or at room temperature.

Almond crêpes with avocado & nectarines

Ingredients

• 2 large eggs

* 3 tbsp ground almonds

* 2 tsp rapeseed oil

* 1 avocado, halved, stoned and flesh lightly crushed

* 2 ripe nectarines, stoned and sliced

* seeds from 1/2 pomegranate

* ½ lime, cut into 2 wedges, for squeezing over

Instructions

* STEP 1

Beat one egg and 1 1/2 tbsp of the almonds in a small bowl with 1 tbsp water. Heat 1 tsp oil in a large non-stick frying pan over a medium heat and pour in the egg mixture, swirling the pan to evenly cover the base. Cook until the mixture sets and turns golden on the underside, about 2 mins. (There is no need to flip it over.) Turn it out onto a plate and make another one with 1 tbsp water, the remaining egg, oil and almonds.

• STEP 2

Top each crêpe with the avocado, nectarines and pomegranate, and squeeze over the lime at the table.

Millet porridge with almond milk & berry compote

Ingredients

• 340g millet

• 1 litre unsweetened fortified almond milk, plus extra to serve

• few mint leaves, to serve

For the compote

• 90g pitted dates, finely chopped

• 500g frozen mixed fruit (ours was a mixed bag of berries, cherries, currants and strawberries)

• 1 cinnamon stick

Instructions

• STEP 1

For the compote, put the dates in a pan with 150ml water, bring to the boil and stir well so they break down. Tip in the frozen fruit and cinnamon stick and cook over a medium heat, stirring every now and then for a couple of minutes. Don't worry about fully thawing larger fruits, as they will defrost in the residual heat and retain their shape in the compote (if you have large strawberries in the mix, you can halve these as they soften). Leave to cool. Will then keep chilled for up to four days.

• STEP 2

Rinse the millet in a sieve, then tip into a deep, heavy-based saucepan and pour in the almond milk and 350ml water. Put over a low heat and once bubbling, leave to simmer for 10-12 mins, stirring frequently until the millet grains are tender, but nutty.

Serve the porridge with the compote. Add a little extra almond milk to serve with a few mint leaves scattered over.

Berry omelette

Ingredients

• 1 large egg

• 1 tbsp skimmed milk

• 3 pinches of cinnamon

• ½ tsp rapeseed oil

• 100g cottage cheese

• 175g chopped strawberry, blueberries and raspberries

Instructions

• STEP 1

Beat egg with milk and cinnamon. Heat oil in a 20cm non-stick frying pan and pour in the egg mixture, swirling to evenly cover the base. Cook for a few mins until set and golden underneath. There's no need to flip it over.

• STEP 2

Place on a plate, spread over cheese, then scatter with berries. Roll up and serve.

Creamy smoked haddock & saffron kedgeree

Ingredients

• 300g basmati rice

• 50g butter

• 3 hard-boiled eggs, shelled and halved

• 200ml double cream

• 500g naturally smoked haddock, skin removed

• 100ml white wine

• 1tsp cayenne pepper

• pinch saffron strands

• 1 tbsp mild curry powder

• freshly grated nutmeg

• small handful flat-leaf parsley, chopped

• 1 lemon, cut into wedges, to serve

Instructions

• STEP 1

Cook basmati rice, leave to cool. Heat oven to 160C/140C fan/gas 3. Grease a large ovenproof dish with some of the butter. Push the egg yolks through a sieve and roughly chop the whites.

• STEP 2

Gently heat the cream in a frying pan until just below boiling point, then add the fish. Cover and poach for 4 mins. Place the wine in a pan with the saffron and warm to infuse. In a large bowl, mix together the rice, cayenne, curry powder, nutmeg, seasoning, chopped egg whites and saffron-infused wine. Lift the fish out of the cream and flake into the bowl – removing any bones as you find them. Scrape in the cream and gently mix together once more.

• STEP 3

Tip everything into the buttered dish and dot the top with the remaining butter. Bake to heat through for 20 mins, then serve scattered with the parsley and sieved egg yolk, with lemon wedges on the side.

Kale & salmon kedgeree

Ingredients

• 300g brown rice

• 2 salmon fillets (about 280g)

- 4 eggs

- 1 tbsp vegetable oil

- 1 onion, finely chopped

- 100g curly kale, stalks removed, roughly chopped

- 1 garlic clove, crushed

- 1 tbsp curry powder

- 1 tsp turmeric

- zest and juice 1 lemon

Instructions

- STEP 1

Cook the rice following pack instructions. Meanwhile, season the salmon and steam over a pan of simmering water for 8 mins or until just cooked. Keep the pan of water on the heat, add the eggs and boil for 6 mins, then run under cold water.

• STEP 2

Heat the oil in a large frying pan or wok, add the onion and cook for 5 mins. Throw in the kale and cook, stirring, for 5 mins. Add the garlic, curry powder, turmeric and rice, season and stir until heated through.

• STEP 3

Peel and quarter the eggs. Flake the salmon and gently fold through the rice, then divide between plates and top with the eggs. Sprinkle over the lemon zest and squeeze over a little juice before serving.

Cured salmon

Ingredients

• 1 tbsp cracked black pepper

• 75g muscovado sugar

• 60g sea salt flakes

• 1 filleted side of very fresh salmon (about 800g), skin on

For the dill & lemon cream cheese

• 200g full-fat cream cheese, at room temperature

• small bunch of dill, finely chopped

• ½ unwaxed lemon, zested and juiced, plus extra wedges to serve

For the pickle

* 1 small cucumber

* 1 small red onion, finely sliced

* pinch of caster sugar

* 3 tbsp white wine vinegar

To serve

* selection of toasted bagels

* sliced rye bread

* small pot of salmon caviar

* caper berries or capers, drained

Instructions

* STEP 1

Up to four days but at least two days before serving the salmon, mix the pepper, sugar and salt together.

Pat the salmon dry with kitchen paper and run your hands over the flesh to find any stray bones – use tweezers to pull these out, if needed. Lay the salmon in a dish, skin-side down, and pack the salt mix over the flesh. Cover the fish with a board or tray weighed down with a few heavy cans or jars. Transfer to the fridge for at least two days or up to four, turning the fillet about every 12 hrs.

• STEP 2

To make the dill cream cheese, beat all of the Ingredients together and set aside. This can be made up to a day ahead and chilled.

• STEP 3

To make the pickle, cut the cucumber in half lengthways, scoop out the seeds using a spoon, and slice into thin half-moons. Toss the cucumber with the red onion and a generous pinch of salt in a colander, then set aside for 30 mins to soften. Transfer the vegetables to a bowl or jar and top up with the sugar and vinegar. Can be eaten immediately or made up to two days ahead and chilled.

• STEP 4

Lift the salmon out of the curing mixture and wipe off any excess seasoning using kitchen paper. Put the fish on a large serving board and carve into thin slices. Serve with the bagels and rye bread, dill & lemon cream cheese, the pickle, salmon caviar, capers and lemon wedges.

CHAPTER V

NOURISHING LUNCH RECIPES FOR PBC

Slow-Cooker Mediterranean Diet Stew

Ingredients

• 2 (14 ounce) cans no-salt-added fire-roasted diced tomatoes

• 3 cups low-sodium vegetable broth

• 1 cup coarsely chopped onion

• ¾ cup chopped carrot

• 4 cloves garlic, minced

• 1 teaspoon dried oregano

• ¾ teaspoon salt

• ½ teaspoon crushed red pepper

• ¼ teaspoon ground pepper

• 1 (15 ounce) can no-salt-added chickpeas, rinsed, divided

• 1 bunch lacinato kale, stemmed and chopped (about 8 cups)

• 1 tablespoon lemon juice

• 3 tablespoons extra-virgin olive oil

• Fresh basil leaves, torn if large

• 6 lemon wedges (Optional)

Directions

1. Combine tomatoes, broth, onion, carrot, garlic, oregano, salt, crushed red pepper and pepper in a

4-quart slow cooker. Cover and cook on Low for 6 hours.

2. Measure 1/4 cup of the cooking liquid from the slow cooker into a small bowl. Add 2 tablespoons chickpeas; mash with a fork until smooth.

3. Add the mashed chickpeas, kale, lemon juice and remaining whole chickpeas to the mixture in the slow cooker. Stir to combine. Cover and cook on Low until the kale is tender, about 30 minutes.

4. Ladle the stew evenly into 6 bowls; drizzle with oil. Garnish with basil. Serve with lemon wedges, if desired.

Delicious Tomato, Feta & Spinach-Stuffed Portobello Mushrooms

Ingredients

• 3 tablespoons extra-virgin olive oil, divided

• 1 clove garlic, minced

• ½ teaspoon ground pepper, divided

• ¼ teaspoon salt

• 4 portobello mushrooms (about 14 ounces), wiped clean, stems and gills removed

• 1 cup chopped spinach

• ½ cup quartered cherry tomatoes

• ⅓ cup crumbled feta cheese

• 2 tablespoons pitted and sliced Kalamata olives

• 1 tablespoon chopped fresh oregano

Directions

1. Preheat oven to 400 degrees F.

2. Combine 2 tablespoons oil, garlic, 1/4 teaspoon pepper and salt in a small bowl. Using a silicone brush, coat mushrooms all over with the oil mixture. Place on a large rimmed baking sheet and bake until the mushrooms are mostly soft, 8 to 10 minutes.

3. Meanwhile, combine spinach, tomatoes, feta, olives, oregano and the remaining 1 tablespoon oil in a medium bowl. Once the mushrooms have softened, remove from the oven and fill with the spinach mixture. Bake until the tomatoes have wilted, about 10 minutes.

Slow-Cooker Quinoa Salad with Arugula & Feta

Ingredients

• 2 ¼ cups unsalted vegetable stock

- 1 ½ cups uncooked quinoa, rinsed

- 1 cup sliced red onions (from 1 onion)

- 2 garlic cloves, minced (about 2 teaspoons)

- 1 (15.5 ounce) can no-salt-added chickpeas (garbanzo beans), drained and rinsed

- 2 ½ tablespoons olive oil

- ¾ teaspoon kosher salt

- 2 teaspoons fresh lemon juice (from one lemon)

- ½ cup drained, chopped roasted red bell peppers (from jar)

- 4 cups baby arugula (about 4 ounces)

- 2 ounces feta cheese, crumbled (about 1/2 cup)

- 12 pitted kalamata olives, halved lengthwise

• 2 tablespoons coarsely chopped fresh oregano

Directions

1. Stir together the stock, quinoa, onions, garlic, chickpeas, 1/2 tablespoon olive oil and 1/2 teaspoon salt in a 5- to 6-quart slow cooker. Cover and cook on LOW until the quinoa is tender and the stock is absorbed, 3 to 4 hours.

2. Turn off the slow cooker. Fluff the quinoa mixture with a fork. Whisk together the lemon juice and remaining 2 tablespoons olive oil and 1/4 teaspoon salt. Add the olive oil mixture and red bell peppers to the slow cooker; toss gently to combine. Gently fold in the arugula. Cover and let stand until the arugula is slightly wilted, about 10 minutes. Sprinkle each serving evenly with the feta cheese, olives and oregano.

Baked Penne Florentine

Ingredients

• 8 ounces dried multigrain or whole wheat penne pasta

• 1 (10 ounce) package frozen chopped spinach, thawed and well drained

• ¼ cup vegetable broth

• 1 medium onion, chopped

• 2 cloves garlic, minced

• ½ cup raw cashews

• 1 ¾ cups water

• 1 15 to 16-ounce can Great Northern beans, navy beans, or cannellini (white kidney beans), rinsed and drained

- 2 teaspoons lemon juice

- ½ teaspoon dry mustard

- ¼ teaspoon salt

- ¼ teaspoon ground black pepper

- ½ cup soft whole wheat bread crumbs

Directions

1. Preheat oven to 375 degrees F. Cook the pasta according to package instructions. Drain and return to hot pan. Add spinach; toss to combine. Spoon into a 2-quart casserole; set aside.

2. In a small saucepan combine vegetable broth, onion, and garlic. Bring to boiling; reduce heat. Simmer, uncovered, about 5 minutes or until onion is tender. Remove from heat and set aside.

3. Place cashews in a food processor. Cover and process until finely ground. Add half of the water and blend until smooth. Add onion mixture, beans, lemon juice, mustard, salt, and pepper. Cover and process until smooth. Transfer to a medium bowl and stir in the remaining water. Stir bean mixture into pasta mixture in casserole. Sprinkle with bread crumbs.

4. Bake, uncovered, about 30 minutes or until crumbs are toasted. Let stand for 10 minutes before serving.

Mediterranean Tuna Antipasto Salad

Ingredients

• 1 15- to 19-ounce can beans, such as chickpeas, black-eyed peas or kidney beans, rinsed

• 2 5- to 6-ounce cans water-packed chunk light tuna, drained and flaked (see Note)

• 1 large red bell pepper, finely diced

• ½ cup finely chopped red onion

• ½ cup chopped fresh parsley, divided

• 4 teaspoons capers, rinsed

• 1 ½ teaspoons finely chopped fresh rosemary

• ½ cup lemon juice, divided

• 4 tablespoons extra-virgin olive oil, divided

• Freshly ground pepper, to taste

• ¼ teaspoon salt

• 8 cups mixed salad greens

Directions

1. Combine beans, tuna, bell pepper, onion, parsley, capers, rosemary, 1/4 cup lemon juice and 2 tablespoons oil in a medium bowl. Season with pepper. Combine the remaining 1/4 cup lemon juice, 2 tablespoons oil and salt in a large bowl. Add salad greens; toss to coat. Divide the greens among 4 plates. Top each with the tuna salad.

Spinach Ravioli with Artichokes & Olives

Ingredients

• 2 (8 ounce) packages frozen or refrigerated spinach-and-ricotta ravioli

• ½ cup oil-packed sun-dried tomatoes, drained (2 tablespoons oil reserved)

• 1 (10 ounce) package frozen quartered artichoke hearts, thawed

• 1 (15 ounce) can no-salt-added cannellini beans, rinsed

• ¼ cup Kalamata olives, sliced

• 3 tablespoons toasted pine nuts

• ¼ cup chopped fresh basil

Directions

1. Bring a large pot of water to a boil. Cook ravioli according to package instructions. Drain and toss with 1 tablespoon reserved oil; set aside.

2. Heat the remaining 1 tablespoon oil in a large nonstick skillet over medium heat. Add artichokes and beans; sauté until heated through, 2 to 3 minutes.

3. Fold in the cooked ravioli, sun-dried tomatoes, olives, pine nuts and basil.

Caprese Stuffed Portobello Mushrooms

Ingredients

• 3 tablespoons extra-virgin olive oil, divided

• 1 medium clove garlic, minced

• ½ teaspoon salt, divided

• ½ teaspoon ground pepper, divided

• 4 portobello mushrooms (about 14 ounces), stems and gills removed

• 1 cup halved cherry tomatoes

• ½ cup fresh mozzarella pearls, drained and patted dry

• ½ cup thinly sliced fresh basil

• 2 teaspoons best-quality balsamic vinegar

Directions

1. Preheat oven to 400 degrees F.

2. Combine 2 tablespoons oil, garlic, 1/4 teaspoon salt and 1/4 teaspoon pepper in a small bowl. Using a silicone brush, coat mushrooms all over with the oil mixture. Place on a large rimmed baking sheet and bake until the mushrooms are mostly soft, about 10 minutes.

3. Meanwhile, stir tomatoes, mozzarella, basil and the remaining 1/4 teaspoon salt, 1/4 teaspoon pepper and 1 tablespoon oil together in a medium bowl. Once the mushrooms have softened, remove from the oven and fill with the tomato mixture. Bake until the cheese is fully melted and the tomatoes have wilted, about 12 to 15 minutes more. Drizzle each mushroom with 1/2 teaspoon vinegar and serve.

Vegan Pesto Spaghetti Squash with Mushrooms & Sun-Dried Tomatoes

Ingredients

• 1 2 1/2- to 3-pound spaghetti squash, halved lengthwise and seeded

• 4 tablespoons extra-virgin olive oil, divided

• 8 ounces cremini mushrooms, sliced

• ½ cup julienned sun-dried tomatoes

• ½ teaspoon salt, divided

• 1 cup packed fresh basil leaves

• 2 cloves garlic, coarsely chopped

• ⅓ cup unsalted raw cashews

• 3 tablespoons lemon juice

• 2 teaspoons nutritional yeast

• ½ teaspoon ground pepper

Directions

1. Place squash halves, cut-side down, in a microwave-safe dish; add 2 tablespoons water. Microwave, uncovered, on High until tender, 10 to 14 minutes. (Alternatively, place squash halves, cut-side down, on a rimmed baking sheet. Bake in a 400 degrees F oven until tender, 40 to 50 minutes. You can also cook the squash in a pressure cooker/multicooker; see Tip.)

2. Meanwhile, heat 1 tablespoon oil in a large skillet over medium heat. Add mushrooms, tomatoes and 1/4 teaspoon salt; cook, stirring, until the mushrooms are soft and starting to brown, 5 to 6 minutes. Remove from heat.

3. Combine basil, the remaining 3 tablespoons oil, garlic, cashews, lemon juice, nutritional yeast, the remaining 1/4 teaspoon salt and pepper in a food processor. Process until mostly smooth.

4. Use a fork to scrape the squash flesh from the shells into a colander. Press lightly on the flesh to remove some of the liquid. Divide the squash among 4 plates. Top each serving with mushroom mixture and then a dollop of basil pesto.

Pesto Pasta Salad

Ingredients

• 8 ounces whole-wheat fusilli (about 3 cups)

• 1 cup small broccoli florets

• 2 cups packed fresh basil leaves

• ¼ cup pine nuts, toasted

• ¼ cup grated Parmesan cheese

• 2 tablespoons mayonnaise

• 2 tablespoons extra-virgin olive oil

• 2 tablespoons lemon juice

• 1 large clove garlic, quartered

• ¾ teaspoon salt

• ½ teaspoon ground pepper

• 1 cup quartered cherry tomatoes

Directions

1. Bring a large saucepan of water to a boil. Add fusilli and cook according to package instructions. One minute before the pasta is done, stir in

broccoli. Cook for 1 minute, then drain and rinse under cold running water to stop further cooking.

2. Meanwhile, place basil, pine nuts, Parmesan, mayonnaise, oil, lemon juice, garlic, salt and pepper in a mini food processor. Process until almost smooth. Transfer to a large bowl. Add the pasta and broccoli, along with tomatoes. Toss to coat.

Spice-cured tuna tacos

Ingredients

For the fish

• 400g fresh line-caught tuna

• 3 tbsp olive oil

• 2 limes, zested, 1 juiced

• 1 tbsp cumin seeds

- 1 tbsp coriander seeds

- ½ tsp chilli flakes

For the avocado purée

- 3 ripe avocados, de-stoned and peeled

- 3 tbsp coriander leaves

- 1 tbsp pickle liquor from the pickled jalapeño chillies

To serve

- 8small soft flour tacos

- vegetable oil, for brushing and drizzling

- pickled jalapeño chillies

- 50g pomegranate seeds

* 1bunch coriander, chopped, with a few leaves left whole

* 4 shredded spring onions

* 2 limes, cut into wedges

Directions

* STEP 1

Slice the tuna into 1cm strips, then dice into rough 1cm cubes. Drizzle over the olive oil and scatter over the lime zest, stir and put in the fridge for 20 mins or so. Gently toast the cumin and coriander in a small frying pan, then tip into a pestle and mortar with a pinch of salt and the chilli flakes and crush to a coarse powder. Stir the spice mix into the tuna with the lime juice and put the bowl back in the fridge for at least 10 mins or up to 1 hr.

* STEP 2

To make the avocado purée, put all the Ingredients in a food processor with a pinch of salt and blitz until you have a smooth purée, adding a little oil if it's too thick to blitz. Spoon the mixture into a container.

• STEP 3

If you like your tacos crispy, heat oven to 180C/160C fan/gas 4, brush them with a little oil, place on a baking sheet and cook for 10-15 mins. To build each taco, spoon on some avocado purée and spread out to the edge. Spoon on the spiced tuna and sprinkle over the chillies, pomegranate seeds, coriander and spring onions, drizzle with more oil and add a lime wedge to the plate. Eat with your hands, if soft, or a knife and fork if crispy.

Cheesy seafood bake

Ingredients

- 300g medium potatoes (about 3), thinly sliced

- 2 tbsp milk

- 40g mature cheddar, finely grated

- 1 tsp rapeseed oil

- 1 onion (160g), finely chopped

- 1 red pepper, deseeded and finely diced (270g)

- 2 tsp balsamic vinegar

- 1 tsp vegetable bouillon powder

- 400g can chopped tomatoes

* ½ x 30g pack basil, leaves picked and finely chopped

* 1 garlic clove, finely grated

* 280g pack skinless cod loins

* 100g frozen small Atlantic cooked prawns, defrosted

* 160g broccoli florets

Directions

* STEP 1

Boil the potato slices for 10 mins then drain, tip into a bowl and gently mix in the milk and half the cheese. Don't worry if the potatoes break up a little.

* STEP 2

Meanwhile, heat the oil in a large frying pan and cook the onion until softened. Stir in the pepper and cook for 5 mins more. Spoon in the balsamic vinegar and bouillon powder, then stir in the tomatoes, basil and garlic. Lay the cod fillets on top, then cover and cook for 6-8 mins until the cod flakes when tested. Heat the grill to high.

• STEP 3

Take off the heat, stir in the prawns and tip into a shallow baking dish, breaking up the cod into large chunks. Cover with the potatoes and sprinkle with the remaining cheese. Grill until golden. While it's grilling, steam or boil the broccoli to serve with the bake.

BBQ mackerel

Ingredients

• 3 tbsp extra-virgin olive oil

• 4 small whole mackerel, gutted and cleaned

For the drizzle

• 1 large red chilli, deseeded and finely chopped

• 1 small garlic clove, finely chopped

• small knob fresh root ginger, finely chopped

• 2 tsp honey

• 2 limes, zested and juiced

• 1 tsp sesame oil

• 1 tsp Thai fish sauce

Directions

• STEP 1

Light the barbecue and allow the flames to die down until the ashes have gone white with heat. Make the drizzle by whisking 2 tbsp olive oil and all the other Ingredients together in a small bowl, adjusting the ratio of honey and lime to make a sharp sweetness. Season to taste.

• STEP 2

Score each side of the mackerel about 6 times, not quite through to the bone. Brush the fish with the remaining oil and season lightly. Barbecue the mackerel for 5-6 mins on each side until the fish is charred and the eyes have turned white. Spoon the drizzle over the fish and allow to stand for 2-3 mins before serving.

Korean fishcakes with fried eggs & spicy salsa

Ingredients

For the fishcakes

• 4 x loch trout or rainbow trout fillets, skinned and cut into 1cm/ 1/2in pieces (about 450g/1lb fish)

• 2 tsp finely grated ginger

• 1 fat garlic clove, crushed

• 1 tsp light soy sauce

• bunch spring onions, thinly sliced

• 1 large egg white, beaten until frothy

• 2 tbsp rice flour

• 2 ½ tbsp vegetable oil, for frying

For the salad

• 1 pointed or small white cabbage, cored and finely shredded (about 350g/12oz)

• 100g radishes, thinly sliced

• 2 tbsp Chinese rice vinegar

• 1 tbsp sesame oil, plus 2 tsp to serve

• 1 tsp gochujang, plus 2 top to serve (see tip)

• 1 tsp golden caster sugar

• 1 garlic clove, crushed

• 2 tsp light soy sauce

• 4 medium eggs

• 1 tbsp sesame seeds, toasted

• 1 red chilli, finely sliced, to serve (optional)

Directions

• STEP 1

For the fishcakes, mix the fish with the ginger, garlic, soy and half the spring onions. Stir in the egg white and rice flour.

• STEP 2

Toss the cabbage and radishes with the vinegar, 1 tbsp sesame oil, 1 tsp gochujang, the sugar and garlic. Set aside. Stir together the remaining sesame oil, gochujang and the soy sauce to make a drizzling sauce for later.

• STEP 3

Heat 1 tbsp oil in a large, non-stick frying pan. Split the fish mixture into eight, then spoon four into the pan, pressing the mix to make cakes about 8cm across. Fry for 2 mins each side until just cooked through and golden. Add another 1 tbsp oil to the pan and repeat with the remaining fish. Keep warm in a low oven.

• STEP 4

Add the remaining oil to the pan. Fry the eggs for 2-3 mins until crisp but with a runny yolk. Serve the fishcakes with the cabbage, and top with the egg and sesame seeds. Scatter with the rest of the spring onions, red chilli (if using) and some of the chilli sesame drizzle.

Classic lasagne

Ingredients

• 2 olive oil, plus extra for the dish

• 750g lean beef mince

• 90g pack prosciutto

• 800g passata or half our basic tomato sauce

• 200ml hot beef stock

• nutmeg

• 300g fresh lasagne sheets

• white sauce (find a recipe in the Directions, or use shop-bought)

• 125g ball mozzarella, torn into thin strips

Directions

• STEP 1

To make the meat sauce, heat 2 tbsp olive oil in a frying pan and cook 750g lean beef mince in two batches for about 10 mins until browned all over.

• STEP 2

Finely chop 4 slices of prosciutto from a 90g pack, then stir through the meat mixture.

• STEP 3

Pour over 800g passata or half our basic tomato sauce recipe and 200ml hot beef stock. Add a little grated nutmeg, then season.

• STEP 4

Bring up to the boil, then simmer for 30 mins until the sauce looks rich.

• STEP 5

Heat the oven to 180C/160C fan/gas 4 and lightly oil an ovenproof dish (about 30 x 20cm).

• STEP 6

Spoon one third of the meat sauce into the dish, then cover with some fresh lasagne sheets from a

300g pack. Drizzle over roughly 130g ready-made or homemade white sauce.

• STEP 7

Repeat until you have three layers of pasta. Cover with the remaining 390g white sauce, making sure you can't see any pasta poking through.

• STEP 8

Scatter 125g torn mozzarella over the top.

• STEP 9

Arrange the rest of the prosciutto on top. Bake for 45 mins until the top is bubbling and lightly browned.

Haddock in tomato basil sauce

Ingredients

• 1 tbsp olive oil

• 1 onion, thinly sliced

• 1 small aubergine, about 250g/9oz, roughly chopped

• ½ tsp ground paprika

• 2 garlic cloves, crushed

• 400g can chopped tomato

• 1 tsp dark or light muscovado sugar

• 8 large basil leaves, plus a few extra for sprinkling

• 4 4x175g/6oz firm skinless white fish fillets, such as haddock

Directions

• STEP 1

Heat the olive oil in a large non-stick frying pan and stirfry the onion and aubergine. After about 4 minutes the vegetables will start to turn golden but won't be soft yet, so cover with a lid and let the vegetables steam-fry in their own juices for 6 minutes – this helps them to soften without needing to add any extra oil.

• STEP 2

Stir in the paprika, garlic, tomatoes and sugar with ½ tsp salt and cook for another 8-10 minutes, stirring, until onion and aubergine are tender.

• STEP 3

Scatter in the basil leaves then nestle the fish in the sauce, cover the pan and cook for 6-8 minutes until the fish flakes when tested with a knife and the flesh is firm but still moist. Tear over the rest of the basil and serve with a salad and crusty bread.

Antipasti salmon

Ingredients

• 100g sundried tomatoes in oil, drained and finely chopped

• small handful of basil, finely chopped, plus a few whole basil leaves

• small handful of dill, finely chopped, plus a few dill fronds to serve

• 2 tbsp capers, drained and rinsed

• 2 garlic cloves, crushed

• 1 lemon, zested and sliced

• 150g butter, softened

• 600g side of salmon, descaled and pin bones removed

• 3 tbsp pitted black olives

• 100g griddled artichoke hearts, drained and roughly chopped

Directions

• STEP 1

Put the tomatoes, half the herbs, 1 tbsp capers, the garlic, lemon zest and butter in a bowl and mash together with a spoon. Alternatively, tip into a food processor and blitz until combined. The flavoured butter will keep, chilled, for up to two days.

• STEP 2

Layer a sheet of baking parchment large enough to loosely wrap the salmon over an equally-sized sheet of foil. Place the salmon on top, then cut the fish into portions, without cutting all the way through to the skin, so the fillet remains intact. Make the portions as big or small as you like, depending on how many you're feeding. Spread the flavoured butter over the salmon, then top with the remaining capers, the lemon slices, olives and artichokes. Wrap the foil and parchment over the salmon and scrunch the ends to seal, creating a loose parcel.

• STEP 3

To bake the salmon, heat the oven to 200C/180C fan/gas 6. Put the parcel on a baking tray and cook for 30 mins, then leave to stand for a few minutes before unwrapping. Alternatively, light the barbecue, wait for the flames to die down, put the parcel directly on the grill and cook for 8-15 mins, or until the salmon is cooked through. Check the salmon is cooked by pushing the flesh with a fork – it should easily flake. Serve on a platter, scattered

with the remaining herbs and the buttery juices
poured over.

CHAPTER VI

NOURISHING DINNER RECIPES FOR PBC

Cheesy leek & potato pie

Ingredients

• 3 leeks, cut into chunks

• small knob butter

• pinch dried rosemary or thyme

• 450g potato (1 very large baking potato is perfect), chopped into thick slices

• 140g melting cheese, such as cheddar, cut into small chunks

• 500g pack shortcrust pastry

• 1 egg, beaten

Instructions

• STEP 1

Put the leeks, butter and herbs in a pan, cover and cook over a low heat for about 20 mins until very soft, stirring occasionally. While the leeks are cooking, put the potatoes in a pan of cold water, bring to the boil and simmer for 4-5 mins until just cooked. Drain the potatoes and stir into the cooked leeks. Leave to cool, stir in the cheese and season with plenty of pepper and salt if you want. The filling can now be chilled for use the following day, if you like.

• STEP 2

Heat oven to 200C/fan 180C/gas 6. Divide the pastry in two and roll one of the pieces to the size of a dinner plate. Transfer this to a baking sheet and roll the remaining pastry and any trimmings to a round about 5cm bigger than the first. Pile the filling into the middle of the round on the baking sheet, leaving a 4cm border. Brush the border with the beaten egg, then drape over the larger piece of pastry. Trim the edges to neaten, then press the sides together with your thumb. Brush the tart all over with egg. Bake for 35-40 mins until golden. Leave to rest for 10 mins before cutting into wedges and serving with beans or greens.

Spring tabbouleh

Ingredients

• 6 tbsp olive oil

* 1 tbsp garam masala

* 2 x 400g cans chickpeas, drained and rinsed

* 250g ready-to-eat mixed grain pouch

* 250g frozen peas

* 2 lemons, zested and juiced

* large pack parsley, leaves roughly chopped

* large pack mint, leaves roughly chopped

* 250g radishes, roughly chopped

* 1 cucumber, chopped

* pomegranate seeds, to serve

Instructions

* STEP 1

Heat oven to 200C/180C fan/ gas 6. Mix 4 tbsp oil with the garam masala and some seasoning. Toss with the chickpeas in a large roasting tin, then cook for 15 mins until starting to crisp. Tip in the mixed grains, peas and lemon zest. Mix well, then return to the oven for about 10 mins until warmed through.

• STEP 2

Transfer to a large bowl or platter, then toss through the herbs, radishes, cucumber, remaining oil and lemon juice. Season to taste and scatter over the pomegranate seeds. Any leftovers will be good for lunch the next day.

Spinach & halloumi salad

Ingredients

• 250g halloumi cheese

* 200g bag spinach

* 2 large oranges

* 1 bunch mint, leaves only

Instructions

* STEP 1

Slice the halloumi and griddle for 3-4 mins each side until charred, then set aside. Tip the spinach and half the mint onto a large platter. Segment the oranges and pour any orange juice from the chopping board into a bowl, and squeeze the pith to get juices from there too. Scatter the orange pieces over the spinach. Chop the remaining mint and mix with the orange juice, 2 tbsp olive oil and some seasoning. Place the halloumi slices on top of the salad and pour the dressing over. Serve with warm flatbreads.

Healthier treacle sponge

Ingredients

- 2 tbsp rapeseed oil, plus ¼ tsp

- 5 tbsp golden syrup

- 1 small orange (½ tsp finely grated zest and 2 tbsp plus 1 tsp juice)

- 175g self-raising flour

- 1 ½ tsp baking powder

- 100g light muscovado sugar

- 25g ground almond

- 2 large eggs

- 175g natural yogurt

• 1 tsp black treacle

• 25g butter, melted

Instructions

• STEP 1

Heat oven to 180C/160C fan/gas 4. Brush 6 x 200ml pudding tins with the ¼ tsp oil, then sit them on a baking tray. Stir together 4 tbsp of the golden syrup, the orange zest and 2 tbsp orange juice and spoon a little into the bottom of each tin (step 1).

• STEP 2

Tip the flour, baking powder, sugar (breaking up any lumps with your fingers) and ground almonds into a large mixing bowl and make a dip in the centre. Beat the eggs in a separate bowl, then stir in the yogurt and treacle. Pour this mixture, along with the melted butter and remaining 2 tbsp oil, into the dry mixture (step 2) and stir together briefly with a large metal spoon, just so everything is well combined. Divide the mixture evenly between the tins (step 3). Bake for 20-25 mins or until the puddings have risen to the top of the tins and feel firm.

• STEP 3

Mix together the remaining 1 tbsp golden syrup and 1 tsp orange juice to drizzle over as a sauce. To serve, if the pudding tops have peaked slightly, slice off to level so they sit upright when turned out. Loosen around the sides with a round-bladed knife (step 4), then turn them out onto plates. Scrape out any syrupy bits remaining in the tins and put on top of the puddings, then drizzle a little of the syrup sauce over and around each one.

Tomato & thyme cod

Ingredients

• 1 tbsp olive oil

• 1 onion, chopped

• 400g can chopped tomatoes

• 1 heaped tsp light soft brown sugar

• few sprigs thyme, leaves stripped

• 1 tbsp soy sauce

• 4 cod fillets, or another white flaky fish, such as pollock

Directions

• STEP 1

Heat 1 tbsp olive oil in a frying pan, add 1 chopped onion, then fry for 5-8 mins until lightly browned.

• STEP 2

Stir in a 400g can chopped tomatoes, 1 heaped tsp light soft brown sugar, the leaves from a few sprigs of thyme and 1 tbsp soy sauce, then bring to the boil.

• STEP 3

Simmer 5 mins, then slip 4 cod fillets into the sauce.

• STEP 4

Cover and gently cook for 8-10 mins until the cod flakes easily. Serve with baked or steamed potatoes.

Creamy salmon, leek & potato traybake

Ingredients

- 250g baby potatoes, thickly sliced

- 2 tbsp olive oil

- 1 leek, halved, washed and sliced

- 1 garlic clove, crushed

- 70ml double cream

- 1 tbsp capers, plus extra to serve

- 1 tbsp chives, plus extra to serve

- 2 skinless salmon fillets

- mixed rocket salad, to serve (optional)

Directions

- STEP 1

Heat the oven to 200C/180C fan/gas 6. Bring a medium pan of water to the boil. Add the potatoes and cook for 8 mins. Drain and leave to steam-dry in a colander for a few minutes. Toss the potatoes with ½ of the oil and plenty of seasoning in a baking tray. Put in the oven for 20 mins, tossing halfway through the cooking time.

• STEP 2

Meanwhile, heat the remaining oil in a frying pan over a medium heat. Add the leek and fry for 5 mins, or until beginning to soften. Stir through the garlic for 1 min, then add the cream, capers and 75ml hot water, then bring to the boil. Stir through the chives.

• STEP 3

Heat the grill to high. Pour the creamy leek mixture over the potatoes, then sit the salmon fillets on top. Grill for 7-8 mins, or until just cooked through.

Serve topped with extra chives and capers and a salad on the side, if you like.

Crushed new potato fish cakes with horseradish mayonnaise

Ingredients

• 750g new potato, cut into large chunks

• 100g baby spinach

• 2 smoked haddock fillets, about 600g

• 700ml whole milk

• 2 bay leaves

• ½ tsp black peppercorns

• 1 egg yolk

• 2 tbsp vegetable oil

• 25g plain flour

• lemon wedges, to serve

For the horseradish mayo

• 250ml mayonnaise

• 50g fresh horseradish, grated (or from a jar)

• juice and zest ½ lemon

Directions

• STEP 1

Cook the potatoes in boiling salted water for 10-15 mins until tender. Drain in a colander over the spinach so the leaves wilt. Return the potatoes to the pan to steam-dry, then roughly crush with a fork. Leave to cool.

• STEP 2

In a separate pan, poach the haddock in the milk with the bay leaves and peppercorns for 4 mins. Turn off the heat and leave to cook for a few mins more until the flesh flakes. Remove to a plate and break into large pieces, discarding the skin and any bones.

• STEP 3

Mix the cooled potato, wilted spinach and haddock with the egg yolk and 3 tbsp of the poaching milk. Form into 4 chunky cakes and chill in the fridge, covered, for at least 30 mins, or overnight. Mix all the mayonnaise Ingredients together and chill.

• STEP 4

Heat the oil in a large pan over a medium heat. Sprinkle flour over the fish cakes and fry for about 5-6 mins on each side until golden and heated through. Serve with lemon wedges and a dollop of the horseradish mayo.

Spicy Singaporean fish

Ingredients

• 2 red chillies, deseeded and chopped

• 2 shallots, chopped

• 1 garlic clove, chopped

• 1 lemongrass, outer leaves removed, chopped

• small knob ginger peeled and chopped

• 2 tsp soy sauce

• pinch sugar

• 2 tbsp vegetable oil

• 2 fillets lemon sole, about 120g each

• chives and coriander, to serve

Directions

• STEP 1

Make a paste by blending together the chillies, shallots, garlic, lemongrass, ginger, soy sauce and sugar in a blender or coffee grinder, or use a pestle and mortar. Heat the oil in a small frying pan and cook the paste for 2 mins until it has darkened slightly and you can really smell the spices. Season with a little salt if you like, then set aside.

• STEP 2

Heat the grill to medium. Put the fish onto a grill pan, then use the back of a teaspoon to smear the paste all over, making a thin layer covering the whole fish. Pop under the grill and cook for 10 mins until the fish flakes easily. Serve with rice and steamed bok choy. Sprinkle chives and coriander on the fish to serve, if you like.

Spiced fish & mussel pie

Ingredients

• 750g parsnip, peeled, cored and cut into large chunks

• 500g potatoes, peeled and cut into medium-sized chunks

• 85g butter

• 300ml fresh fish stock

• 1kg fresh mussel, scrubbed clean

• 1 large onion, chopped

* 1 tbsp medium curry powder or paste

* 50g plain flour

* 400ml can coconut milk

* 750g Icelandic cod fillet, skinned and cut into large cubes

* 100g cooked tiger prawns

* 1 pack fresh coriander, chopped

Directions

* STEP 1

Boil the parsnips and potatoes for 15-20 mins until tender. Drain and mash well with 25g/1oz butter and seasoning. Cover and set aside.

* STEP 2

Bring the stock to the boil in a large pan. Tip in the mussels, cover and leave to steam for about 3 mins, or until the shells open. Drain into a colander set over a large bowl to reserve the stock. Remove and throw away the shells and any un-opened mussels. Cover the cooked mussels to stop them drying out.

• STEP 3

Melt the remaining butter and fry the onion until softened. Stir in the curry powder and fl our, and cook for about 1 min. Pour in the coconut milk and 3-4 tbsp of the reserved mussel stock and stir well until you have a smooth sauce. Leave to simmer for 5 mins until thickened.

• STEP 4

Add the cod to the sauce, return to a simmer and cook for 3-4 mins, stirring occasionally, but trying not to break up the cod. Stir in the mussels, prawns and coriander, season, then tip into a large ovenproof dish. Spread the parsnip mash over the top.

• STEP 5

To serve now heat the grill and grill until the mash is golden and crusty. To eat later cool, cover, then chill for a couple of hours. To serve, heat oven to 200C/ fan 180C/gas 6 and bake for 35-40 mins until hot all the way through.

Spicy fish cakes with mango dipping sauce

Ingredients

• 1kg medium-sized floury potato such as Maris Piper, unpeeled

• 10 tbsp vegetable oil

- 2 tsp mustard seed

- 2 tbsp curry leaf, fresh or dried

- 2 red onions, finely chopped

- 2 red chillies, deseeded and chopped

- 50g ginger, finely chopped

- zest 1 lemon

- 2 eggs, lightly beaten

- 600g skinless salmon fillet

- 250g skinless smoked haddock

- 300ml milk

For the coating

- 6 tbsp plain flour, seasoned

• 3 eggs, lightly beaten

• 200g fresh white breadcrumb

For the mango dipping sauce

• 4 tbsp mango chutney

• juice 2 limes

• 2 tbsp shredded mint

Directions

• STEP 1

Put the potatoes in a large saucepan, cover with salted water, bring to the boil and cook until tender. Drain, leave to cool, then peel and mash.

• STEP 2

Heat 4 tbsp of the oil in a pan set over a medium heat. Add the mustard seeds, half the curry leaves, onions, red chillies and ginger, and fry for 5 mins until the onions have softened. Add onion mixture to the mashed potato with the lemon zest, mix well, then work in the eggs.

• STEP 3

Put the salmon and smoked haddock in a pan. Add the remaining curry leaves, then pour over the milk plus enough water to cover. Put on the lid and simmer for 3-4 mins, then turn off the heat and leave the fish in the pan for 10 mins to finish cooking. Take the fish out of the milk and leave to cool. Using your hands, break into big flakes, add to the potato mixture and mix gently to combine.

• STEP 4

Shape mixture into patties about 9cm diameter and 3cm thick. For the coating, dust each with flour, then dip into the egg and coat with breadcrumbs.

Transfer to a tray lined with baking parchment and chill for 30 mins. The fish cakes can be frozen at this point. Put the tray in the freezer and when frozen, pop the fish cakes in bags and seal.

• STEP 5

Heat the remaining oil in a frying pan and cook the fish cakes, in batches, for 7-8 mins each side, until golden and crisp. Drain on kitchen paper. To cook fish cakes from frozen, see below.

• STEP 6

Combine all the dipping sauce Ingredients and stir in 4-5 tbsp water to thin it down. Serve with the fish cakes.

One-pan Thai green salmon

Ingredients

• 2 tbsp vegetable oil

• 2 shallots, thickly sliced

• 1 green chilli, deseeded if you like, and sliced, plus extra to serve

• 300g baby new potatoes, quartered

• 1 lemongrass stalk, bashed

• 4 tbsp Thai green curry paste

• 400g can coconut milk

• 200-300ml vegetable stock

• 1-2 tbsp fish sauce

• ½-1 tbsp brown or palm sugar

• 1 courgette, trimmed and peeled into ribbons

• 100g baby spinach

• 4 skinless salmon fillets

• 3 limes, 2 juiced plus 1 cut into wedges to serve

• 3 spring onions, finely sliced (optional)

• handful of coriander or Thai basil, roughly chopped, to serve

• cooked jasmine rice or rice noodles, to serve (optional)

Directions

• STEP 1

Heat the oven to 200C/180C fan/ gas 6. Put the oil in a deep roasting tin or dish about 30 x 25cm and toss through the shallots, chilli, potatoes and lemongrass. Roast for 10 mins until fragrant, keeping an eye on the shallots to ensure they don't burn. Remove from the oven and stir in the curry paste to coat everything. Return to the oven for 2 mins until its aroma is released before mixing in the coconut milk and 200ml stock. Put back in the oven again for 15-20 mins until the sauce is slightly thickened and the potatoes are turning tender.

• STEP 2

Season to taste with the fish sauce and sugar, then stir through the courgette ribbons and spinach. Add another 50ml-100ml stock now if the sauce is too thick, but be aware that the courgette and spinach will release some water as well. Nestle the salmon fillets in the sauce and bake for a further 10-15 mins until the salmon is cooked to your liking.

• STEP 3

Add the lime juice and taste the sauce for a balance of sweet and sour, adding more lime juice and fish sauce, if you like. Scatter over the spring onions, if using, along with the herbs and chilli. For a more filling meal, serve with rice or noodles and the lime wedges on the side.

Indian-spiced fish cakes

Ingredients

- 600g potato, quartered if large

- ½ tsp cumin seeds

- 2 spring onions, finely chopped

- 1 red chilli, deseeded and finely chopped

- 2 tbsp chopped coriander

- 1 egg, beaten

- 100g cooked leftover salmon, flaked into large pieces

• plain flour, for coating

• 25g butter and 1 tbsp sunflower oil

• leftover avocado mayo, raita or mango chutney, to serve

Directions

• STEP 1

Boil the potatoes. Meanwhile, dry-fry the cumin seeds for a couple of secs in a large non-stick frying pan. When soft, drain the potatoes, return to the saucepan, add the cumin, onions, chilli and coriander with plenty of seasoning, then mash well. When cooled a little, beat in 2 tbsp of the egg, then carefully stir through the salmon. Shape into 4 rough cakes, then coat in flour. If freezing, freeze on a baking sheet until solid, then pack up.

• STEP 2

In the frying pan, melt the butter with the oil. Fry the cakes for about 2 mins each side until golden. Serve with the mayo, raita (recipe below) or mango chutney and some salad leaves.

Tomato & mascarpone risotto

Ingredients

• 2 tbsp olive oil

• 1 onion, very finely chopped

• 1 large garlic clove, crushed

• 175g risotto rice

• 400g can cherry tomatoes

• 600ml hot vegetable stock

• 30g parmesan or vegetarian alternative, grated

• 30g mascarpone, or cream cheese

• ½ small bunch of basil, chopped

Directions

• STEP 1

Heat the oil in a large, heavy-based saucepan. Add the onion along with a pinch of salt, and fry for 10 mins or until beginning to soften and turn translucent, then add the garlic and fry for 1 min. Stir in the rice and cook for 2 mins.

• STEP 2

Tip in the tomatoes and bring to a simmer. Add half the stock, cooking and stirring until absorbed. Add the remaining stock, a ladleful at a time, and cook until the rice is al dente, stirring constantly for around 20 mins.

• STEP 3

Stir through the parmesan, mascarpone or cream cheese, and basil, then season to taste. Spoon into bowls to serve.

Mustard salmon & veg bake with horseradish sauce

Ingredients

• 4 parsnips, sliced lengthways

• 4 small raw beetroot, thickly sliced

• 6 carrots, sliced lengthways

• 2 tbsp olive oil

• 4 x 125g/4½oz pieces salmon with skin

• 2 tbsp grainy mustard

* 2 tbsp hot horseradish

* 150ml crème fraîche

* 1 tbsp cider vinegar

* 1 tbsp chopped dill

Directions

* STEP 1

Heat oven to 200C/180C fan/gas 6. Toss all the vegetables with the oil and season well. Spread in a single layer on 2 baking trays (or 1 very large tray) and roast for 30 mins.

* STEP 2

Season the salmon and spread over the mustard. In the final 10 mins of cooking the veg, add the salmon to the trays.

• STEP 3

In a small bowl, mix together the horseradish, crème fraîche, vinegar, dill and some seasoning. Serve the salmon with the sauce and veg.

Hake fish cakes with mustard middles

Ingredients

For the fish cakes

• 450g floury potatoes, cut into chunks (we used Rooster potatoes)

• 1 bay leaf

• a few peppercorns

• 450g skinless hake fillet, cut into 4

• bunch spring onions, finely shredded

- 1 whole nutmeg

- 3 tbsp plain flour, seasoned

- 1 egg

- 100g fresh breadcrumbs

- 2l vegetable oil, for deep-frying

- salad leaves, to serve

- lemon wedges, to serve

For the mustard middles

- 100g full-fat crème fraîche

- 50g strong cheddar, grated

- 1 egg yolk (reserve the white)

- 1 tbsp wholegrain mustard

Directions

• STEP 1

Mix all the mustard middle Ingredients together. Drape cling film across a muffin tin, then spoon the mix into 4 of the wells. Freeze for 30 mins or until solid.

• STEP 2

Put the potatoes, bay leaf and peppercorns in a pan of cold water, bring to the boil and cook for 20 mins or until tender. Remove and allow to steam-dry in a colander. Add the fish to the water and simmer for 5 mins until it is just cooked through at the thickest part.

• STEP 3

Mash the potatoes and stir in the spring onions, a little freshly grated nutmeg and some seasoning.

Drain the hake, then flake it into the mash. Gently mix everything together and leave to cool.

• STEP 4

Divide the fish mixture into 4. Shape 1 fish cake at a time, moulding it into a ball. Make a well in the centre of the ball and push a frozen mustard middle into it, then shape the mash around it to make a smooth hockey-puck shape. Repeat with the remaining fish, then freeze for 15 mins.

• STEP 5

Using 3 shallow bowls, add the flour to one; put the egg and reserved egg white in another, and the breadcrumbs in the third. Beat the eggs with some seasoning. Thoroughly coat the fishcakes first in the flour, then the egg , then the breadcrumbs. Freeze the fish cakes until firm. Can be frozen for up to 1 month – defrost in the fridge for 2 hrs before cooking.

• STEP 6

When ready to cook, heat the oil to 180C in a large, deep saucepan (or use a fat fryer) and the oven to 190C/170C fan/gas 5. Fry the fish cakes for 7 mins, turning halfway, until crisp. Drain on kitchen paper, transfer to a baking sheet and bake for 5 mins (15 mins from frozen) so the middles are hot. Serve with dressed leaves and a lemon wedge.

Baked sea bream with tomatoes & coriander

Ingredients

• 4 large potatoes, about 1kg/2lb 4oz

• 2 garlic cloves, finely chopped

* pinch dried chilli flakes

* pinch saffron

* 1 bunch coriander, roughly chopped

* 4 whole sea bream, cleaned and gutted

* 1 tbsp olive oil, plus extra for greasing

* juice 2 limes

* 125ml white wine

* handful sundried tomatoes

* handful pine nuts, toasted

* 4 thin slices pancetta or smoked streaky bacon

Directions

* STEP 1

Heat the oven to 200C/180C fan/gas 6. Slice the potatoes thinly, put in a large saucepan and cover with cold salted water. Bring to the boil and drain, then lay onto the base of a lightly oiled large baking tray. Scatter over the garlic, chilli, saffron and a little of the coriander.

• STEP 2

Slash the fish through the flesh down to the bone – this allows it to cook evenly and quicker than normal. Season and rub with the olive oil. Lay the fish on the potatoes and top with the lime juice, wine, tomatoes and pine nuts. Lay the pancetta slices over the fish and bake for 20-25 mins or until the fish is cooked through. Check by pulling out one of the fins on the back, it should come away easily. Serve the fish scattered with the remaining coriander.

CHAPTER VII

NOURISHING SIDE DISH RECIPES FOR PBC

Cheesy roasted courgettes

Ingredients

• 4 courgettes, halved lengthways

• 250g tub ricotta

• zest 1 lemon

• 1 chilli, deseeded and finely chopped

• handful chopped herbs, such as mint, parsley and basil

• 4 tbsp dried breadcrumbs

Directions

• STEP 1

Heat oven to 200C/180C fan/gas 6. Use a teaspoon to scoop the seeds from the middle of each courgette half, then place them in a large baking tray.

• STEP 2

Mix together the ricotta, zest, chilli and herbs, and season with salt and pepper. Pile the stuffing into the courgettes and top with breadcrumbs. Bake for 35 mins until the courgettes are tender and the topping is golden and crisp.

Baked feta with sesame & honey

Ingredients

• 1 tbsp sesame seeds, toasted

• 200g block feta

• 2 tbsp honey, plus extra to serve

• 1 tsp roughly chopped oregano

• olive oil, for drizzling

• warmed pitta breads, to serve

Directions

• STEP 1

Heat the oven to 200C/180C fan/gas 6, or if using an air-fryer, heat to 180C for 3 mins. Put the sesame seeds in a shallow dish and brush the block of feta all over with the honey. Carefully press the honey-coated feta into the sesame seeds, turning so that it's well crusted with seeds.

• STEP 2

Put the feta in a baking dish (it should fit snugly), then sprinkle over the oregano and a pinch of sea salt. Drizzle with some olive oil. Bake in the oven for 15-20 mins, or cook in the air-fryer for 15 mins until the feta is soft, then drizzle with a little extra honey and serve with the pitta breads on the side.

Smoked haddock & cheddar fishcakes with watercress sauce

Ingredients

• 425g floury potatoes, cut into large chunks

• 1 bay leaf

• 6 peppercorns

• small bunch flat-leaf parsley, leaves and stalks separated

• 225g smoked haddock fillets, skin on (we used dyed haddock to give the mash a lovely golden colour)

• 200g unsmoked haddock fillets, skin on

• 75g mature British cheddar, grated

• 4 spring onions, 0.5 very finely sliced, 0.5 roughly chopped

• 50g plain flour

• 2 medium eggs, beaten

• 100g fresh breadcrumbs

• sunflower oil, for frying

• 50g watercress (weighed after discarding the thickest stalks)

• 4 tbsp rapeseed oil

• 2 lemons, 1 juiced, 1 cut into small wedges to serve (optional)

Directions

• STEP 1

Put the potatoes, bay leaf, peppercorns and parsley stalks in a big pan of cold water. Cover with a lid, bring to the boil and cook for 15 mins until tender. Using a slotted spoon, transfer the potatoes to a colander and leave to steam-dry. Turn the heat down, add the fish and poach gently for 5 mins until it flakes easily. Tip the potatoes into a big bowl and put the fish in the colander to drain for a few mins.

• STEP 2

Add the cheese, some pepper and a little salt to the potatoes and mash well. Flake in about half the fish, discarding the skin and bones, and mash in too. Flake in the remaining fish in big chunks, scatter over the sliced spring onions and gently mix together. Roll the mixture into golf-ball-sized cakes.

• STEP 3

Tip the flour onto a plate and season. Tip the egg and breadcrumbs into 2 shallow bowls each. Roll each fishcake first in the flour, then the egg, then the breadcrumbs. Sit on some parchment-lined trays that fit in your fridge. Chill for at least 1 hr or up to 24 hrs.

• STEP 4

Fill a deep frying pan with 1-2cm of sunflower oil, heat until shimmering, then brown a few fishcakes at a time, turning regularly. If the oil gets too crumby, change halfway through. You can serve them straight away, or cool and chill for up to 24 hrs in the fridge, then simply warm for 30 mins in an oven at 180C/160C fan/ gas 4 before the party.

• STEP 5

Make the dipping sauce up to 1 hr before serving – put the roughly chopped spring onions, the parsley leaves, watercress, rapeseed oil, 2 tbsp lemon juice and 5 tbsp water in a food processor or blender. Whizz to the consistency of single cream.

• STEP 6

Pile the warm fishcakes onto a platter with a bowl of watercress sauce on the side and some lemon wedges for squeezing over, if you like.

Lemon & coriander couscous

Ingredients

* 250g couscous

* grated zest of a lemon

* 2 x 20g packs fresh coriander

* 4 tbsp raisins

* 4 tbsp toasted pine nuts

Directions

* STEP 1

Prepare 250g couscous with boiling water or stock, according to the packet's instructions.

* STEP 2

Add the lemon zest, fresh coriander, raisins and pine nuts. Season well and drizzle with plenty of olive oil. Goes really well with fish or lamb.

Perfect roast potatoes

Ingredients

• 16 potatoes the best ones to use are Desirée, as they hold their shape, but King Edward and Maris Piper are also good

• 2 tbsp plain flour

• 140g goose fat or duck fat or dripping

• 3 tbsp sunflower oil or vegetable oil

Directions

• STEP 1

Heat oven to 190C/fan 170C/gas 5. Peel the potatoes and cut in half; if very large, cut into quarters, or leave whole if they are small. Tip into a saucepan, cover with cold water, then bring to the boil. Set the timer and boil for exactly 2 mins. Drain the potatoes well, then toss in the colander to fluff up their surfaces, sprinkling over the flour as you go.

• STEP 2

Place a large, sturdy roasting tray over a fairly high heat, then tip in the fat and oil. When sizzling, lower in the potatoes carefully, then gently brown in the hot fat for about 5 mins so all the sides are covered with oil.

• STEP 3

Roast undisturbed for 20 mins, then remove from the oven and gently turn them over with a fish slice. Place the tray on the hob to heat the oil, then return to the oven and cook for another 20 mins. Turn again, putting the tray back on the hob to heat the oil. Give them a final 20 mins in the oven, by which time you should have perfect roast potatoes.

Courgette & anchovy salad

Ingredients

• ¼ tsp fennel seed

• juice and zest ½ lemon

• 1 tbsp extra-virgin olive oil, plus extra for drizzling

• 1 garlic clove, crushed

• 1 large courgette, thinly sliced on the diagonal

• 50g rocket

• 2 anchovy fillets, halved

Directions

• STEP 1

Toast the fennel seeds in a small frying pan over a low-medium heat for 1 min, or until they release their aroma. Bash them lightly using a pestle and mortar. Mix the lemon juice, fennel seeds, oil and garlic in a large bowl, then stir in the courgette. Season and set aside to marinate for 30 mins.

• STEP 2

Toss through the rocket and transfer to a platter. Top with the anchovy fillets. Scatter with lemon zest and serve with an extra drizzle of olive oil.

Barbecued fennel with black olive dressing

Ingredients

• 2 fennel bulbs, sliced lengthways into 1cm-thick pieces

• 1 ½ tbsp olive oil

• 2 tbsp finely chopped black Kalamata olive

• 1 garlic clove, crushed

• juice 1 lemon

• small handful each parsley and basil, finely chopped

Directions

• STEP 1

Heat a BBQ or griddle pan. Toss the fennel in 1 tbsp of the oil, coating well. Cook for 5 mins on each side until golden brown and charred.

• STEP 2

To make the dressing, put the olives, garlic, lemon juice and remaining oil in a bowl. Add the chopped herbs and combine. Lay the fennel on a platter and pour over the dressing. Eat warm or at room temperature.

Apricot pancakes with honey butter

Ingredients

For the butter

• 100g butter, softened

• 2 tbsp clear honey

For the pancakes

• 140g self-raising flour

• pinch bicarbonate of soda

• 25g caster sugar

• 1 egg

• 150ml milk

• handful ready-to-eat dried apricots, finely chopped

• oil, for frying

Directions

• STEP 1

For the honey butter, beat the butter with the honey and spoon onto a large piece of cling film. Squeeze into a sausage shape, then wrap tightly and chill until ready to use. Will keep in the fridge for up to a month.

• STEP 2

Sift the flour, bicarbonate of soda and a small pinch of salt into a bowl, then stir through the sugar and make a well in the centre. Beat together the egg and milk, then gradually pour into the well, stirring slowly, to avoid creating lumps. Stir in the apricots.

• STEP 3

Heat a non-stick frying pan over a low heat and add a little oil. Drop in 4 tablespoonfuls of batter and cook for 1 min or until the surface of each pancake is covered in bubbles. Flip with a palette knife or fish slice, then cook for a further min. Repeat with the remaining batter. Serve warm or leave to cool, then toast and spread with the honey butter to serve

Harissa cauliflower pilaf

Ingredients

- 300g basmati rice

- 1 red onion, finely sliced

- 2 lemons, 1 juiced, 1 cut into wedges

- 2 tsp sugar

- 4 tbsp harissa

- 1 garlic clove, crushed

- 1 tbsp olive oil

- 1 large or 2 medium cauliflower, broken into large florets, stalk chopped, large leaves roughly chopped

- pinch of saffron

- 2 bay leaves

- 700ml hot vegan vegetable stock

- 100g sultanas

• 100g flaked almonds, toasted until golden brown

• ½ small bunch of dill, chopped, plus extra to serve

• 400g can chickpeas, drained and rinsed

• 50g pomegranate seeds (optional)

Directions

• STEP 1

Wash the rice really well, then leave to soak in cold water for 1 hr. Put the onion in a small bowl and toss with the lemon juice, the sugar and a pinch of salt. Leave to pickle while you make the pilaf.

• STEP 2

Heat the oven to 200C/180C fan/gas 6. Whisk 2 tbsp harissa, the garlic and oil in a large bowl, then add the cauliflower and toss to coat in the sauce. Season, then tip into a roasting tin and roast for 30 mins until tender and golden.

• STEP 3

Meanwhile, mix the saffron, bay leaves, stock and 2 tbsp harissa in a pan over a very low heat to keep warm while the cauli roasts.

• STEP 4

Remove the cauli from the oven, tip into a dish and squeeze over the juice from one of the lemon wedges. Drain the rice and tip into the roasting tin. Pour over the infused stock, and mix well. Stir in the sultanas, half the almonds, the dill, chickpeas, and half the cauliflower. Cover the tin with a double layer of foil, sealing well, then bake for 30 mins until the rice is tender and stock is absorbed.

• STEP 5

Fluff up the rice with a fork, then fold in the remaining cauliflower (this creates a contrast of cauli textures). Scatter over the extra dill, the remaining almonds, the pomegranate seeds, if using, the pickled red onions and remaining lemon wedges to squeeze over.

Quinoa, pea & avocado salad

Ingredients

• 100g frozen peas

• juice 1 lemon

• 2 tbsp olive oil

• ½ small pack mint, leaves only, chopped

• ½ small pack chives, snipped

• 250g pack ready-to-eat red & white quinoa mix (we used Merchant Gourmet)

• 1 avocado, stoned, peeled and chopped into chunks

• 75g bag pea shoots

Directions

• STEP 1

Put the peas in a large heatproof bowl, pour over just-boiled water, then set aside.

• STEP 2

Pour the lemon juice into a small bowl and whisk in some seasoning. Keep whisking as you slowly add the olive oil, followed by the mint and chives.

• STEP 3

Drain the peas and tip into a large serving dish. Stir in the quinoa, breaking up any clumps. Pour over the dressing, then fold in the avocado and pea shoots. Serve immediately.

Spicy salmon tabbouleh

Ingredients

• 400g bulgur wheat

• 500g salmon fillet, pin-boned

• 3 tbsp sunflower oil

• 2 onions, finely chopped

• 5cm piece ginger, peeled and finely chopped

• 2 tbsp curry paste (we used korma)

• 300g Greek yogurt

• juice 1 lemon, plus 2 cut into wedges, to serve

• 300g smoked salmon

• handful coriander or parsley, roughly chopped

Directions

• STEP 1

Cook the bulgur wheat in plenty of salted water for 7 mins (or follow pack instructions). Drain, tip into a large bowl and leave to cool. Put the salmon fillet on a foil-lined grill, brush lightly with oil and season. Grill for 7-10 mins, turning halfway, until the fish flakes easily. Cool.

• STEP 2

Heat the remaining oil, add the onions and ginger, and fry for about 5 mins until softened and lightly coloured. Stir in the curry paste and cook for 1 min, stirring. Remove from the heat and stir in the yogurt, lemon juice and some seasoning. Leave to cool.

• STEP 3

Skin and flake the salmon fillet. Cut the smoked salmon into strips. Add the fresh salmon and half the smoked salmon to the bulgur wheat with the dressing and half the coriander. Stir everything together lightly, so as not to break up the salmon flakes too much. Tip onto a serving platter and scatter over the remaining smoked salmon strips and coriander. Add the lemon wedges and serve.

Warm mackerel & beetroot salad

Ingredients

• 450g new potato, cut into bite-size pieces

• 3 smoked mackerel fillets, skinned

• 250g pack cooked beetroot

• 100g bag mixed salad leaves

• 2 celery sticks, finely sliced

• 50g walnut pieces

For the dressing

• 6 tbsp good-quality salad dressing

• 2 tsp creamed horseradish sauce

Directions

• STEP 1

Boil the potatoes for 12-15 mins until just tender. Meanwhile, flake the mackerel fillets into large pieces and cut the beetroot into bite-size chunks.

• STEP 2

Drain the potatoes and cool slightly. Mix the salad dressing and horseradish sauce together in a salad bowl and season. Tip in the potatoes – they should still be warm.

• STEP 3

Add the salad leaves, mackerel, beetroot, celery and walnuts, and toss gently. Serve with crusty bread.

Courgettes with mint & ricotta

Ingredients

• 2 tbsp olive oil

• 2 tsp unsalted butter

• 4 large courgettes (we used a mixture of green and yellow), sliced

• zest and juice 1 lemon

• pinch of chilli flakes

• 70g ricotta

• extra virgin olive oil, for drizzling

• handful mint leaves, picked and roughly chopped

Directions

• STEP 1

Heat a large, heavy non-stick frying pan or cast-iron skillet over a medium heat. Heat 1 tbsp of the oil and 1 tsp butter together and add half the courgettes in one layer. Cook for 2 mins, then turn the heat down to medium-low and cook for 5 more mins untouched, until the underside has a nice colour. Flip the courgettes, then grate over some lemon zest, pour over half the lemon juice and season with salt, pepper and chilli flakes. Cook for a further 5 mins or until very tender. Repeat the process with the remaining slices of courgette.

• STEP 2

Transfer to a platter and top with spoonfuls of ricotta. Drizzle over some extra virgin olive oil and scatter over the mint to serve.

Stir-fried greens with fish sauce

Ingredients

• ½ head Savoy cabbage

• 125g purple sprouting or Tenderstem broccoli

• 2 tbsp groundnut oil

• 4-6 garlic cloves, finely sliced

• 75g baby spinach

• 2 tbsp fish sauce, plus extra for seasoning

• 1 tsp caster sugar

Directions

• STEP 1

Remove any discoloured or coarse leaves from the cabbage, then halve it. Remove the hard central ribs and discard them, then shred the leaves. If using purple sprouting broccoli, halve any thicker stems lengthways.

• STEP 2

Heat the oil in a wok. Stir-fry the broccoli for 1 min, then add the garlic and cabbage and cook until the garlic is a pale gold colour. Quickly add the spinach and fish sauce and turn the veg over – the moisture should come out of the spinach and boil off quickly. Add the sugar and toss the vegetables again, then add a little more fish sauce, if you like.

Fish o'leekie

Ingredients

• 1 leek, finely sliced

• 500ml vegetable stock

• 300g basmati rice

• 500g cod or haddock fillet, skinned and cut into large chunks

• handful parsley, roughly chopped

• finely grated zest and juice 1 lemon

Directions

• STEP 1

Put the leek in a large microwave dish with 4 tbsp
of the stock. Cover the dish with cling film, pierce
the film with a knife, then microwave on High for 5
mins.

• STEP 2

Uncover the dish, then stir the rice and remaining
stock into the leek. Re-cover with cling film, pierce
and microwave on High for another 10 mins,
stirring halfway through until the rice is very nearly
cooked.

• STEP 3

Gently stir in the fish chunks, cover the dish with
cling film again, then pierce and cook for a further
5 mins until the fish flakes easily and the rice is
tender. Stir in the parsley, lemon zest and juice.
Leave to stand for 2 mins before serving.

CHAPTER VIII

BEFORE YOU LEAVE, A FINAL WORD!

Lifestyle and home remedies

You may feel better if you take good care of your overall health. Here are some things you can do to improve some primary biliary cholangitis symptoms and, possibly, help prevent certain complications:

• **Choose reduced-sodium foods**. Sodium adds to tissue swelling and to the buildup of fluid in your abdomen. Look for low-sodium foods or naturally sodium-free foods.

• **Avoid eating oysters or other raw shellfish.** Such seafood can carry infection-causing bacteria. Infections can be dangerous for people with liver disease.

• **Exercise most days of the week.** Exercise may reduce your risk of bone loss.

• **Don't smoke**. If you don't smoke, don't start. If you currently smoke, talk with a healthcare professional about strategies to help you quit.

• **Avoid alcohol.** Your liver processes the alcohol you drink. The added stress can cause liver damage. Generally, people with primary biliary cholangitis should not drink alcohol.

• **Check with your healthcare team before starting new medicines or dietary supplements.** Because your liver isn't working normally, you'll likely be more sensitive to the effects of medicines and some dietary supplements. Check with your healthcare team before taking anything new.

Coping and support

Living with an ongoing liver disease with no cure can be frustrating. Fatigue alone can have a large impact on your quality of life. Each person finds ways to cope with the stress of an ongoing disease. In time, you'll find what works for you. Here are some ways to get started:

• **Learn about your condition.** The more you understand about primary biliary cholangitis, the more active you can be in your own care. In addition to talking with your healthcare team, look for information at your local library and on websites affiliated with reputable organizations such as the American Liver Foundation.

• **Take time for yourself**. Eating well, exercising and getting enough rest can help you feel better. Try to plan ahead for times when you may need more rest.

• **Get help**. If friends or family want to help, let them. Primary biliary cholangitis can be exhausting, so accept the help if someone wants to do your grocery shopping, wash a load of laundry or cook your dinner. Tell those who offer to help what you need.

• **Seek support**. Strong relationships can help you maintain a positive attitude. If friends or family have a hard time understanding your illness, you may find that a support group can be helpful.

Caring for Your Emotional and Mental Health

The first step in taking care of your mental and emotional health is to talk to your primary care doctor. They may refer you to a mental health professional.

Also, focus on things that bring you joy, like watching your favorite TV show or going for a walk. If you still feel anxious, take 15 minutes out of each day for "worry time." Just be sure it's not close to the time you go to bed. Use this time to think about all your worries and even write them down. Then set them aside and come back to the present moment.

Resources and Support for PBC Patients

You can find more information on primary biliary cholangitis from:

American Liver Foundation

National Institute of Diabetes and Digestive and Kidney Diseases

National Organization for Rare Disorders

www.ingramcontent.com/pod-product-compliance
Lightning Source LLC
Chambersburg PA
CBHW061037250726
48653CB00001B/140